BIOSTATS

DATA ANALYSIS FOR DENTAL HEALTH CARE PROFESSIONALS

By Weintraub, Douglass & Gillings

Second Edition

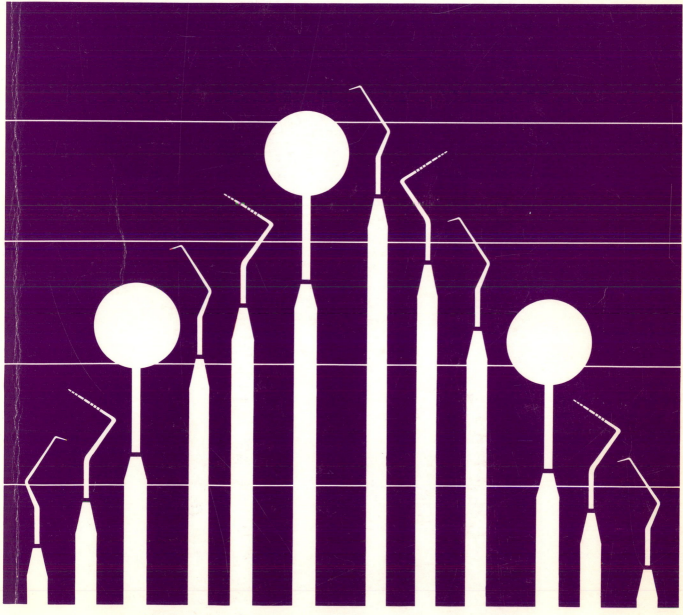

BIOSTATS

DATA ANALYSIS FOR DENTAL HEALTH CARE PROFESSIONALS

In Collaboration with

Marilie Gammon, MSPH
Research Epidemiologist
Department of Dental Care Administration
Harvard School of Dental Medicine

Anila Wijesinha, PhD
Research Statistician
Department of Dental Care Administration
Harvard School of Dental Medicine

William Sollecito, DrPH
Biostatistical Director
Quintiles,Inc.
Chapel Hill, North Carolina

182
Gold

Apdc

WITHDRAWN

BIOSTATS

DATA ANALYSIS FOR DENTAL HEALTH CARE PROFESSIONALS

Second Edition

Y 1 0 2

Jane A. Weintraub, DDS, MPH
Assistant Professor
Program in Dental Public Health
School of Public Health
University of Michigan

Chester W. Douglass, DDS, PhD
Associate Professor and Chairman
Department of Dental Care Administration
Harvard School of Dental Medicine

Dennis B. Gillings, PhD
Professor
Department of Biostatistics
School of Public Health
University of North Carolina

1985 CAVCO Inc. Publishing Division of
Quintiles, Inc., Chapel Hill, N.C.

CAVCO Publications   A Division of Quintiles, Inc.
                            1829 East Franklin Street
                            500 Franklin Square
                            Chapel Hill, North Carolina 27514

Library of Congress copyright © by CAVCO, Incorporated under the Uniform Copyright Convention.

All rights reserved. This book is protected by copyright.

No part of this book may be reproduced, stored in a retrieval system, or transmitted in any form by electronic, mechanical, verbal, photocopying, or recording means without the express written permission from the publisher.

Printed in the United States of America by Benjamin Franklin Smith Printers, Boston, Massachusetts.

Library of Congress Cataloging in Publication Data

Weintraub, Jane A., 1954-
    Biostats, data analysis for dental health care
professionals. Second edition.

    Includes bibliographies and index.
    1. Dentistry — Statistical methods.   I. Douglass,
Chester W., 1940-   . II. Gillings, Dennis B.,
1944-   . III. Title. [DNLM: 1. Dentistry.
2. Statistics.   WU 25 W424b]
RK52.45.W45 1985   617.6'0072   85-12797
ISBN 0-932137-01-6

Last digit is the print number 9 8 7 6 5 4 3 2 1

Oversize
RK
52.45
.W45
1985

Acknowledgements

The teaching material that provided the original draft for this book was first formulated in 1973–1974 as individual self-instructional statistics packages by Dennis Gillings with assistance from Neil Smith, R.M. Sievogel, and Roy Kuebler for teaching biostatistics to the medical students at the University of North Carolina. Using these self-instructional packages Jane Weintraub and Chester Douglass, with the statistical supervision of Dennis Gillings, wrote fourteen packages for the Harvard School of Dental Medicine dental students. Since then, Marilie Gammon has contributed the chapter on epidemiology, collaborated as primary co-author of the nonparametric statistics chapter and as contributing co-author of Chapter 11. Anila Wijesinha collaborated as the primary co-author of the analysis of variance and correlation and regression chapters. Over this ten year history, the numbers of graduate students and faculty colleagues who have reviewed and given constructive criticism on each package (or chapter) have been too numerous to name. Several secretaries and prodution assistants have made special contributions; in particular they are: Bea Parker, Debbie Goss, Wendy Redgrave, Jonathan Director and Gwen Litz.

The authors are particularly grateful for the participation of Ellen Marcus Libert in the project. Ms. Libert is responsible for the graphics and layout; her exceptional creativity is illustrated by the "normal distribution of dental instruments" cover design.

Comments on the Second Edition

Several colleagues have provided reviews and criticism on the first edition of this book. We are particularly grateful for the encouragement and comments of Richard MacKenzie of the University of Florida, David Striffler of the University of Michigan and Cathy Berkey of Harvard University. Sara Creagh of Quintiles Corporation in Chapel Hill, North Carolina has been supportive of the production of the new and revised chapters.

Two new chapters have been added in this second edition. William Sollecito has collaborated as a co-author of Chapter 20 on Experimental Designs and Clinical Trials which introduces the major research designs that are becoming increasingly important in evaluating preventive measures, diagnostic tests, and new treatment methods. Chapter 21 responds to the request of many students and colleagues for a guide to writing a research protocol and evaluating research reports that appear in professional journals. A short bibliography of suggested further reading has also been added in this second edition.

We wish to thank Leo and Donna Phalen of Quill Publications for many improvements in the manuscript and Frank Stiriti of Benjamin Franklin Smith Printers in Boston for his expert suggestions and guidance regarding printing and production of this second edition.

August 1985
Jane Weintraub
Chester Douglass
Dennis Gillings

WILLIAM F. MAAG LIBRARY
YOUNGSTOWN STATE UNIVERSITY

Directions to the Reader:

This self-instructional book has been designed to enable you to master the basic concepts of biostatistics and epidemiology that are utilized in dental research and referred to in the dental literature. In the beginning of each chapter a concept is introduced and objectives are listed. Examples pertaining to dentistry are used throughout the text. Some of the examples are based on actual data, in which case the sources of the information are identified. Other examples are fictitious, although any resemblance to actual research is not purely accidental.

In order to obtain the maximum benefit from this educational opportunity, the authors recommend that you try to solve the problems presented in the text as they are encountered, and compare your answers with the correct answers at the end of each chapter before continuing to the next section. If you have difficulty with a particular concept, read through the material again and carefully examine the solutions to the problems. At the end of each chapter is a review section which highlights the important concepts and terminology that has been discussed. After you think that you have an understanding of the material, try to solve the posttest at the end of the chapter. Your instructor has the answers to the posttests for each chapter.

The format used is for self-paced learning. This book can also be used as a quick reference by someone with previous knowledge of statistics, or as an introductory text for a beginner. Suggestions for further reading, related to each of the statistical methods and design issues discussed in this text, are provided within some of the chapters and at the end of Chapter 21.

Take as much or as little time as you require.

Enjoy the course!

TABLE OF CONTENTS

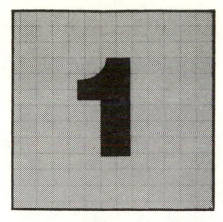

CHAPTER 1

DATA AND TABLES

INTRODUCTION

Dental care providers as clinicians, scientists, teachers, managers and policy makers, must understand and use statistical principles every day. The minimum requirement is the ability to critically read the scientific and professional literature. The clinical scholar, however, must master the fundamentals of statistical logic and be able to apply the basic principles of research design, statistical inference and probability.

This instructional chapter is the first of a series of chapters designed to teach you several basic concepts and techniques in biostatistics. Each chapter is self contained, although some of the later ones require knowledge of earlier chapters in the series.

The first topic is the presentation of descriptive data which is an important area since the statistical principles outlined in this and the next two chapters cover many of the ideas and methods used to understand and communicate different types of data.

OBJECTIVE

You will be able to construct a table that describes a given data set.

BASIC TERMINOLOGY

Data exist in many forms. They may be in the form of symbols, as for example, grades for a course being recorded as a letter of the alphabet, or they may be in numerical form. Generally, to give meaning to "raw data" it is necessary to arrange them into mutually exclusive categories according to some type of scale. There are four different types of scales available: nominal, ordinal, interval and ratio.

In a **nominal scale**, the discrete categories do not have a quantitative relationship to each other. Examples of a nominal scale would be to record the results of an examination as pass/fail, or the answers to a question as yes/no.

In an **ordinal scale**, the categories can be ranked in an increasing or decreasing order. However, the amount of difference between categories is not specified. The use of A, B, C letter grades is an example of an ordinal scale. Unless specific numerical quantities are assigned to each letter, the difference between an A and a B is not necessarily the same as the difference between a B and a C.

In an **interval scale**, the categories are arranged in equally spaced units and the relative difference between each point on the scale can be measured. There is no absolute zero point. A Centigrade thermometer is an example of an interval scale. The difference between 30°C and 31°C is the same as 82°C and 83°C. However, 100°C is not twice as hot as 50°C.

Age is an example of a **ratio scale**. There is an absolute zero point (birth), and the magnitude of differences between ages is the same. Thus, David who is 18 is twice as old as his brother Michael who is 9. An examination in which the lowest possible score is zero and the highest score is 100 is another example of a ratio scale.

DATA SETS

Since research data usually consist of several numbers organized in some way, we will refer to each number as an **item of data** and the totality of items as a **data set**. For example, if the grades that a student received in a head and neck anatomy course were listed, the results might be: 85, 92, 94, 89, 95. Each of these numbers is an item of data and the five items comprise the data set.

Problem 1:
Dental students were screening patients in a clinic and making the following diagnoses: no obvious need for treatment; some treatment needed; substantial amount of treatment needed; treatment needed as soon as possible.

What type of scale are they using?

Your Solution:

Problem 2:
Suppose you counted the number of missing teeth in the next six geriatric dental patients you treated and recorded the numbers as follows: 8, 12, 16, 10, 14 and 21 missing teeth/person.

Using the terminology we have just developed, how would you refer to this group of six numbers, and what type of scale do these counts of missing teeth represent?

Your Solution:

(Solutions are given at the end of the chapter)

Now we can start thinking about how we might describe data. Perhaps the most common method which is used in the majority of scientific papers is to present data items in a table such as the following.

Table 1.1

FIRST-YEAR STUDENTS IN DENTAL SCHOOLS
Academic Years 1970-71 Through 1977-78

Academic Year	SEX		Total: First-year Students
	Male Students	Female Students	
1970-71	4,471	94	4,565
1971-72	4,598	147	4,745
1972-73	5,113	224	5,337
1973-74	5,054	391	5,445
1974-75	4,986	631	5,617
1975-76	5,056	707	5,763
1976-77	5,133	802	5,935
1977-78	5,074	880	5,954
Total	**39,485**	**3,876**	**43,361**

SOURCE: American Dental Association, Council on Dental Education, *Annual Report on Dental Education, 1977-78.*

Table 1.1, as all tables, consists of several standard parts:

1. Title
The title is best kept short and identifies the data items that are found in each cell of the body of the table. In Table 1.1 these data items are the number of "First Year Students in Dental Schools."

2. Headings
a) The **spanner heading** for the variable represented by the columns is simply "Sex" in this example.
b) **Column headings** usually consist of the mutually exclusive and exhaustive categories of the column spanner heading. Obviously, there are only two sex categories — male and female — in this example.
c) The **row category heading** is found to the left of the column spanner heading and identifies the variable that makes up the rows. In Table 1.1, "Academic Year" is the row category heading.
d) **Row labels** are then used to identify the components of the category heading.
e) **Totals** are often used for both the row and column variables. The total values are sometimes called "marginals" because, as you can see, they are found at the right hand and bottom margins of the table.
f) The **source** of the data or table is identified in a footnote just under the table if the data are not original with the publication in which it is found.

Suppose you are a practitioner in a solo practice and you have an office staffing problem. You feel that the time is right to look for a second dentist or another dental auxiliary but you are not sure what type of dentist, hygienist, laboratory technician or assistant would best suit the practice. It seems as though you treat a lot of children but you cannot really say how many. Also, you are not sure of the amount of preventive and diagnostic services you provide, or the specialty services that you might be able to refer. You need to know what type of services each age group of patients in the practice receives in order to judge the areas of service with which you need the most help.

As a first step you decide to identify the type of services received by each age group of patients in the practice. You decide that the age groupings < 3, 3-6, 7-12, 13-17, 18-24, 25-44, 45-64 and 65 years and older, are appropriate age groups. You employ a clerk to tabulate all the active patients seen in the practice during the past two years in terms of their age and type of services received.

Problem 3:

How would you illustrate the information collected by the clerk in a table that describes the patient age and type of service of your practice population?

Your Solution:

Your table should be similar to Table 1.4 with a title such as "Number of Services by Age of Patient and Type of Service." The spanner heading is "Age of Patient" with the specific age groups as the column headings that are relevant to the types of personnel you are considering. The row category heading is the "Type of Service" with the major types of services as the row labels. Totals would be convenient as they eliminate arithmetic calculations on the part of the reader, who might want a quick glance at, say, the total number of patients between 7-12 years of age in the practice or a total percentage distribution of the types of services rendered. Thus, the title, row and column headings and row labels help to clarify what the table is describing.

Problem 4:

Once having constructed a table we can use it to examine the data set which it contains. For example, in Table 1.2 you might wish to know the number of patient services the practice delivered to patients who are under 13 years old and over 65 years old. What would be your answer?

Table 1.2

NUMBER OF SERVICES BY AGE OF PATIENT AND TYPE OF SERVICE RENDERED

Type of Service	Age of Patient								
	<3	3-6	7-12	13-17	18-24	25-44	45-65	>65	Total:
Preventive	5	10	24	24	7	42	73	15	200
Diagnostic	4	13	27	26	9	53	95	53	280
Operative	3	25	80	73	21	156	280	163	801
Removable						4	140	108	252
Surgical			10	5	9	12	30	24	90
Fixed					4	118	134	74	330
Endodontics					2	19	37	10	68
Periodontics						6	21	3	30
Orthodontics			7	8					15
Total	**12**	**48**	**148**	**136**	**52**	**410**	**810**	**450**	**2066**

Your Solution:

Reading from a table is fairly straightforward, although it is often tedious to construct a table. If you have a lot of data you may need the aid of a computer. However, for smaller data sets you can create tables by hand. The clerk or business manager who constructed Table 1.2 might have constructed charts, one for each type of service, by checking the age categories for each service while reviewing the total list of the dental records in the dentist's practice (an example of a check list for surgical services is shown here).

Table 1.3

SURGICAL SERVICES

	<3	3-6	7-12	13-17	18-24	25-44	45-65	>65

The active patients must be classified systematically by marking the appropriate column for each patient. A block of five marks is recorded " ⊞." The headings for each category are written at the bottom of the page and blocks are recorded working up the page.

At this stage you should be ready to take the post test. Please be sure you answer this test correctly before moving on to the next chapter.

SOLUTIONS

Problem 1:
This is an example of an ordinal scale.

Problem 2:
If you said *data set* you are right; and the type of scale is a ratio scale because there is a zero point and 16 missing teeth are twice as many as 8 missing teeth.

Table 1.4

Problem 3:

NUMBER OF SERVICES BY AGE OF PATIENT AND TYPE OF SERVICE RENDERED

Type of Service	Age of Patient								Total:
	<3	3-6	7-12	13-17	18-24	25-44	45-65	>65	
Preventive									
Diagnostic									
Operative									
Removable									
Surgical									
Fixed									
Endodontics									
Periodontics									
Orthodontics									
Total									

Problem 4:
The answer is the sum of the first three column totals plus the last total for the 65 column. 12 + 48 + 148 + 450 = 658.

POSTTEST 1

The names and dates of birth of the 55 most active patients in a dentist's practice are listed below. Construct a table describing the age and sex of these patients and describe what you learn about this dental practice from the table. A worksheet is provided on the next page. Assume that you are doing this on January 1, 1992. It might be helpful to first read the two "hints" given below before beginning the Post Test:

1) When computing the age of each patient, it may be helpful to put the age in parentheses beside the dates of birth.
2) Count the number of males and females in the patient list, then you can later perform a quick accuracy check by comparing these totals to their corresponding age-sex blocks.

YOUR ANSWERS TO POSTTEST 1

Name:

Patient's Name	Date of Birth	Sex	Patient's Name	Date of Birth	Sex
Howard Therrell	4/18/30	M	Virginia Howard	2/22/24	F
Joel Patterson	8/29/83	M	Robert Scarborough	9/01/80	M
Leslie Maness	2/12/47	M	Ethel Shumaker	1/15/48	F
William Fleckenstein	7/04/74	M	Pamela McManus	9/14/34	F
Cora Lee Flanders	3/15/53	F	Larry Lovingood	12/03/50	M
Susan Snuggs	11/24/30	F	Len Ludwig	1/12/62	M
Eugene Ghent	1/02/24	M	Patricia Lussardi	10/01/49	F
Lucille Busby	12/19/32	F	Daniel Fitz-Henry	6/20/84	M
Gladys Nesbit	4/10/52	F	Loree Bjorklund	8/24/35	F
Cecil Putnam	7/27/34	M	Wendy Clark	7/14/75	F
Jay Swalchick	5/30/42	M	Janie Grier	1/01/50	F
Anita White	6/13/51	F	Ruth Medlin	12/18/64	F
Sally Cornelius	3/02/28	F	Joyce Parker	2/20/77	F
Lorraine Romano	12/03/61	F	Robin Levine	5/02/22	F
Dick Brooks	12/02/76	M	Susan Fisher	3/19/74	F
Judy Marcus	7/09/77	F	Karen Walter	6/03/21	F
Tom Burbank	1/19/77	M	Marilyn Monahan	7/04/23	F
Debbie Johnson	8/25/82	F	Barbara Bradford	11/08/75	F
Steve Goldman	5/07/84	M	Jan Dooley	7/25/70	F
Mary Hunter	11/25/60	F	Elizabeth O'Brien	6/22/84	F
Barbara Harrison	8/08/20	F	Lee Grant	4/09/75	M
Julia Jacobs	9/05/40	F	Alice Emery	4/17/75	F
Mona Rappaport	6/16/61	F	Mark Fleming	10/05/77	M
Ellen Anderson	9/19/19	F	Katie Ford	5/12/76	F
Nancy Smith	9/18/79	F	Eleanor Friedman	8/06/54	F
Bill Greene	3/11/82	M	Amy Spring	10/27/17	F
Jill Gallagher	5/15/84	F	Linda Phillips	6/10/76	F
Ann Good	9/04/55	F			

WILLIAM F. MAAG LIBRARY
YOUNGSTOWN STATE UNIVERSITY

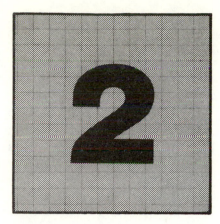

CHAPTER 2

RATES

INTRODUCTION

In the first chapter we considered the construction of tables to describe data. We will now go a stage further with descriptive data and introduce **rates**, which describe the **proportion of individuals with certain attributes within the total population under study**.

For example, insurance companies are interested in the utilization rate for each type of dental service. Suppose you know that 1,000 people in a community visited a dentist during a certain year. The number 1,000 tells you something about those individuals, but does not tell you whether or not the community is utilizing dental services. If the community is of size 2,000, then the use of dental services is about equal to the national average - 50 percent per year. However, if the community consists of 5,000 individuals, you might want to investigate why so few people are receiving dental care.

A rate is really a proportion, and describes the part that possesses a particular attribute compared to the whole. The dental utilization rate may be defined as the proportion of the population that has made a dental visit during the preceding year. For the community of 2,000 with 1,000 making a visit, this would be 1,000/2,000 = 1/2 or 50%.

Problem 1:
What is the rate for the community of 5,000?

Your Solution:

OBJECTIVE

1) After working through this chapter you will be able to define four rates: **incidence, prevalence, sensitivity** and **specificity.**
2) Also, you will be able to compute these rates when given appropriate data.

Problem 2:
Now, without looking back at the preceding definition on this page, what is a rate?

Your Solution:

During the 1980 school year at Walt Whitman High School, which had an enrollment of 2500 students, 20 students suffered from "accidental" injuries to the teeth. These injuries all involved fractured teeth which occurred while the students were playing football or hockey.

Problem 3:
What was the school's dental injury rate for that year?

Your Solution:

In practice, there may be a problem here. A rate is calculated from reported data and if there were several injuries that were not reported, our injury rate would be in error. **Care should be taken to verify the accuracy of reported data.** Also, not all 2500 students were at equal risk of sustaining football or hockey injury. Obviously, only those students who played these sports were at risk. If 120 students were so involved, the dental injury rate for students at risk is 1/6 or 16.7% - a very high rate!

Now, what if you read that during 1980 the six neighboring high schools reported an annual dental injury rate of about 4 percent for contact sports participants? Would this suggest something unique about Walt Whitman High School? Perhaps the athletes are not wearing mouthguards and the local dentists would want to investigate the preventive measures taken by these teams.

INCIDENCE AND PREVALENCE

There are two important rates widely used in epidemiology. They are called incidence rates and prevalence rates and generally refer to the occurrence of disease in a population.

$$\text{Incidence rate} = \frac{\text{Number of new cases of the disease that occur during a given time period}}{\text{Total number of people in the population during the same time period.}}$$

The time period is often one year, but it can be a day, a week, or months when dealing with a rapidly spreading infectious disease. Over an entire year, the population may change due to people moving into or leaving the community of interest. Then the denominator is taken as the average number of people in the population during the year. **Incidence** indicates how many *new* cases of a disease are occurring relative to the total population, but does not say how much of the total disease there is at a given time. This leads us to the definition of **prevalence.**

$$\text{Prevalence rate} = \frac{\begin{array}{c}\text{Number of cases of the disease} \\ \text{existing at a given point in time}\end{array}}{\begin{array}{c}\text{Total number of persons in the} \\ \text{population at that time.}\end{array}}$$

Now read statement A and statement B and answer Problem 4.

Statement A: During October 1981 a team of dentists examined each adult on an Indian reservation in New York State to determine the proportion of adults with enamel defects.

Statement B: A dentist in a hospital practice in Boston counted the number of patients presenting at her office with newly developed hyperkeratotic lesions on the oral mucosa during the month of November, 1981. The dentist also counted the total number of patients in her practice during the same month.

Problem 4:

What rate were the doctors attempting to learn in Statement A? What rate did the dentist tabulate in Statement B?

Your Solution:

SENSITIVITY AND SPECIFICITY

Two other rates which are very useful are sensitivity and specificity. These rates may be used to evaluate a diagnostic test.

Suppose a test is used to classify patients as positive (disease present) and negative (disease absent). It is unlikely that a diagnostic test will be correct every time, and so there will be some patients classified positive who do *not* have the disease (false positives) and other patients classified as negatives who *do* have the disease (false negatives). Now, suppose the population is tested and it is possible to determine by other means (the celebrated "gold standard") if the individuals absolutely do have the disease. Then the population may be classified in the following table:

Table 2.1

TABLE TO EVALUATE A DIAGNOSTIC TEST

	DISEASE STATE	
TEST RESULT	**Disease**	**No Disease**
Positive	True Positives	False Positives
Negative	False Negatives	True Negatives

The **sensitivity** of the diagnostic test is defined as:

$$\text{Sensitivity} = \frac{\text{True Positives}}{\underset{\text{(patients with the disease)}}{\text{True Positives + False Negatives}}} \times 100\%$$

i.e., **the percent of persons with the disease** who are correctly classified as having the disease.

The **specificity** is defined as:

$$\text{Specificity} = \frac{\text{True Negatives}}{\underset{\text{(patients without the disease)}}{\text{True Negatives + False Positives}}} \times 100\%$$

i.e., the **percent of persons without the disease** who are correctly classified as not having the disease.

One way to distinguish between sensitivity and specificity rates is to associate sensitivity with selecting *those who have it,* and specificity with identifying *those who don't have it*. There is an indirect relationship between these two rates that can be visualized in Figure 2.1.

Figure 2.1

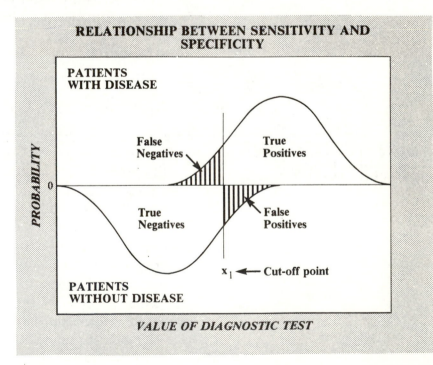

There are two curves, one above the horizontal x-axis, called the abscissa, which represents the distribution of having a certain disease given different values of "x," and one below the x-axis which represents the distribution of the "x" values for patients not having the disease. These "x" values are the results of a diagnostic test such as diastolic blood pressure or white blood count for which a range of values are possible. As you can see from the diagram, there is some overlap between the two curves. At some "x" values for this diagnostic test, there are people who have the disease and some who do not. If a certain cut-off point is selected, as indicated by the solid vertical line labeled "x," then all patients with a test value to the right of the line will be defined as having the disease, and all those to the left of the line will be defined as being disease free. However, those in the shaded part of the "Patients with disease" curve to the left of the x_1 line will be *false negatives*. They really have the disease, but it is not indicated (or predicted) by the result of the test. Those in the shaded part of the "Patients without disease" curve to the right of the x_1 cut-off point will be *false positives*. According to the criteria established by the results of the test, they have been diagnosed as having the disease, when in fact, they really do not. By altering the cut-off point of the test, and moving the location of the vertical line, the sensitivity and specificity of the test is changed.

In Figure 2.2, a smaller value of "x" has been selected as the determining factor in classifying someone as having the disease (i.e., high blood pressure) or not. The line labeled x_2 identifies this new cut-off point.

Figure 2.2

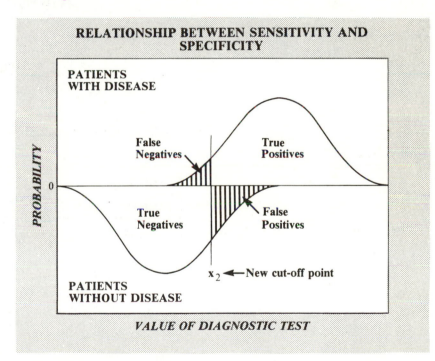

As you can see by the smaller shaded area under the "Patients with disease" curve, this change results in fewer false negatives and more true positives, and thus a greater test sensitivity. However, at the same time, the shaded area associated with the "Patients without disease" curve has increased leading to more false positives and fewer true negatives, which reduce the specificity of this diagnostic test.

The trade-off between sensitivity and specificity will often depend on the risks versus the benefits of *not treating* someone who *has* a disease, in contrast with *treating* someone who *does not have* the disease. Quantitative techniques that fall under the general heading **decision analysis** have been developed which can be applied to the decision to treat or not treat under conditions of uncertainty.

The two rates, sensitivity and specificity, are expressed as percentages. In fact, any percentage is a rate as it is the proportion with an attribute multiplied by 100. Often, rates are expressed as parts of 1,000 or 100,000. Death rates are usually expressed by the number of persons who die in one year per 1,000 population. Morbidity rates by convention are often expressed per 100,000 population.

REVIEW

1) Rate $= \dfrac{\text{Number of individuals with a characteristic}}{\text{Total number of individuals in population}}$

2) Incidence rate $= \dfrac{\text{Number of new cases of the disease that occur during a given time period}}{\text{Total number of persons in the population during the same time period}}$

3) Prevalence rate $= \dfrac{\text{Number of cases of the disease existing at a given point in time}}{\text{Total number of persons in the population at that time}}$

4) Table to evaluate a diagnostic test:

Table 2.2

TEST RESULT	DISEASE STATE	
	Disease	**No Disease**
Positive	True Positives	False Positives
Negative	False Negatives	True Negatives

5) Sensitivity rate *(those who have it)* $= \dfrac{\text{True Positives}}{\text{True Positives + False Negatives}} \times 100\%$

6) Specificity rate *(those who don't have it)* $= \dfrac{\text{True Negatives}}{\text{True Negatives + False Positives}} \times 100\%$

SOLUTIONS

Problem 1:
1,000/5,000 = 1/5 (Why can't life always be this simple?)

Problem 2:
Did you write ... *a proportion which describes that part having a certain attribute, compared to the whole,* or something to that effect? Good.

Problem 3:
20/2500 or 1/125 which is less than 1%.

Problem 4:
In Situation A the doctors were attempting to determine the *prevalence* of enamel defects on the reservation and in Situation B the dentist was trying to determine the *incidence* of hyperkeratosis for the population of patients served by the hospital practice in Boston during the month of November, 1981.

POSTTEST 2

In September, 1983, 200 first year medical and dental students moved into a large dormitory located across the street from the university's medical complex. As part of the orientation to the health sciences center all of the students were required to participate in an oral health examination in the dental school. The resulting dental records indicated that there were 2 cases of students presenting with acute necrotizing ulcerative gingivitis (ANUG). The fall term passed and the students were kept exceedingly busy with their full load of basic science courses. During the week of December 18th, just prior to their first set of final examinations, the university infirmary saw 25 students who complained of painful, sore gums. Examinations were conducted by the attending physician and 10 students were diagnosed as having ANUG and all were referred to the dental school clinic. The periodontists at the dental school, using more specific diagnostic tests and criteria, concluded that only 7 of the 10 students diagnosed as having ANUG, did in fact have this disease, as well as 3 of the additional 15 students that were given a negative report. The other students were suffering from other forms of periodontal disease that have a different pathophysiology. All students were treated accordingly.

1) What was the prevalence of ANUG at the time of the orientation session for the medical and dental students?
2) What was the incidence rate of ANUG during the week of December 18th?
3) Give the sensitivity and specificity rate of the diagnostic examination performed at the infirmary and use the periodontists' definitive diagnosis as the gold standard for separating patients with and without this acute form of periodontal disease.

YOUR ANSWERS
TO POSTTEST 2

Name:

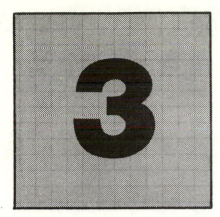

CHAPTER 3

ADJUSTED RATES

INTRODUCTION

Some of the most controversial current topics in dentistry are the perceived trends in the periodontal diseases, dental caries and oral cancer. When you become involved in dental epidemiological research, whether through actual experience or through reading the literature, you will need to compare disease rates for some event or characteristic across different populations. Populations to be compared may be different communities, treatment groups, or two groups — one of which was exposed to a particular disease while the other was not. If the two populations or samples being compared were similarly constituted with respect to factors (such as age, sex, income) that are associated with the event under study, there would be no problem in comparing simple **crude** rates as they stand; however, if the samples or populations are not similarly constituted, a straightforward comparison of crude rates may be misleading.

This chapter is intended to teach you 1) the **conditions** necessary for recognizing such potentially misleading situations and 2) how to statistically cope with such situations through a procedure which will remove the effects of such additional factors (such as age) on the comparison of interest. This procedure is called **rate adjustment.**

In this chapter, you will become familiar with the direct and indirect methods of rate adjustment. We will start by describing when you need to adjust rates.

OBJECTIVE

1) You will be able to state the four conditions necessary for rate adjustment and be able to use these conditions to evaluate whether such adjustment is appropriate.
2) You will be able to use both the direct and indirect methods to adjust rates.

RATE ADJUSTMENT

Briefly examine Figure 3.1 given on the next page, which compares the overall tooth mortality experience of two cities in 1984. Try to get a general feeling for what this illustration is expressing and then go on.

Figure 3.1

A COMPARISON OF NUMBER OF MISSING TEETH IN
TWO CITIES

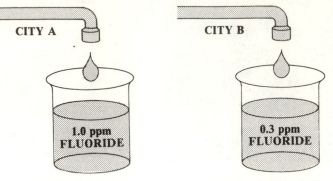

6.9 Missing Teeth/Person   5.3 Missing Teeth/Person

If you were a dental epidemiologist interested in the relationship between concentration of fluoride in the water supply and tooth mortality rate (# missing teeth per person) you might decide to study these two cities, because you could compare the tooth mortality of the population living in an optimally fluoridated area with one that is deficient in fluoride.

The tooth mortality rates for these two cities are:

City A: 953,000 missing teeth/138,000 people = 6.9 missing teeth/person

City B: 462,500 missing teeth/79,500 people = 5.8 missing teeth/person

You might be surprised and a bit confused to find that City A, with its optimal fluoride, has a higher rate of missing teeth per person.

Problem 1:

Which city would you have expected to have had the higher rate, knowing that optimal fluoride levels help to prevent dental caries which can subsequently lead to tooth mortality?

Your Solution:

The next logical question is, "Who lives in these two cities?" A little knowledge of the populations might cause you to adjust your interpretation. Look at the age structures of the two cities in Figure 3.2.

Figure 3.2

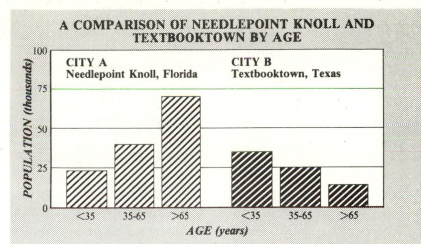

As it turns out, City A is located in a warm climate and a large percent of its real estate is composed of retirement communities. It has tended to attract an older population. On the other hand, City **B** is a newly developed city which has been built up around a large university. It has attracted many younger persons with many children.

What factor associated with tooth mortality rates should cause you to adjust your earlier interpretation of the crude rate? _____

If you answered *age* you are correct because it is likely that the difference in crude rates can be at least partially explained by the simple fact that City A has an older population than City **B**. We should consequently expect relatively more missing teeth in City A simply because there are relatively more people there at high risk of losing their teeth, especially from periodontal disease which becomes more common with increasing age.

The presence of a variable such as **age** in this situation is one of the conditions necessary for computation of adjusted rates. We call such a variable a **confounding factor** because it confounds or blurs the comparison we wanted to make. We initially intended to compare the tooth mortality rates in two cities with different fluoride levels, but unless we also take into account the effects of age, our results might be misleading; therefore, age is a confounding factor making it difficult to ascribe the difference observed in crude tooth mortality rates to the difference in fluoride only.

Problem 2:

The difference that we have observed in crude rates can be explained at least partly by the difference in _____ of the populations and not entirely by differences in _____ between City A and City **B**.

Your Solution:

Problem 3:

The variable *age* in the above example interferes with the comparison of interest (tooth mortality in two cities with different fluoride levels). Therefore, it is a _____ factor in the comparison of the crude tooth mortality rates of City A and City B.

Your Solution:

Problem 4:

If the two crude rates had been exactly the same, this would give some evidence to suggest that the age factor has no effect on overall tooth mortality.

Your Solution:

True _____   False _____

Problem 5:

The existence of a _____ _____ such as age is the primary condition for requiring rate adjustment.

Your Solution:

Now, let's consider all the components of the entire situation. You are faced with a problem that requires **rate adjustment** if the following four conditions pertain:

1) You are interested in a **comparison** of two or more populations or samples.
2) The event or characteristic of interest (in this case, tooth loss) is defined for purpose of analysis as a **rate** (e.g. tooth mortality rate) or **proportion.**
3) Your comparison involves **overall** or crude rates, and
4) There is a **confounding factor** which you feel could affect the comparison.

Figure 3.3

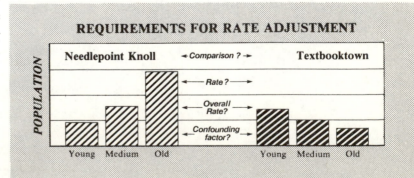

Problem 6:

Check Figure 3.3 to see if all four of the following conditions are satisfied in this case.

a) Do we want to make a comparison? If yes, what is being compared?

b) Is the event of interest defined as either a rate or proportion? If yes, what is the item of interest?

c) Do we want to compare overall rates?

d) Is there a confounding factor? If yes, what is it?

Your Solution:

Problem 7:

If for our example you were *only* interested in comparing the tooth mortality rates for persons in the age group 35-64, would you need to do rate adjustment? Give two reasons for your answer:

Your Solution:

Overall vs. Specific:

With regard to the above question, you should know that some epidemiologists have claimed that you are actually *never* primarily interested in an overall rate. This is a pretty strong attack and deserves some discussion! Let's digress a bit to consider this point of view.

A digression:

An epidemiologist named Woolsey (1959), expressing an opinion shared by several other researchers, has pointed out that "specific rates are essential because it is only through the analysis of specific rates that an accurate and detailed study can be made of the variation among population classes." In the above case, we would analyze the age-specific tooth mortality rate for each age interval and compare the rate obtained for each of the two cities.

Problem 8:

Some epidemiologists claim that you should *never* adjust rates since the only meaningful rates are _____ rates.

Your Solution:

Problem 9:

We certainly agree that specific rates are very important for allowing accurate and detailed analysis. However, we do not agree that the use of _____ rates is *never* appropriate.

Your Solution:

An overall rate can be quite useful as a **convenient summary** of the information in an entire schedule of specific rates. If the influence of a confounding factor is known, it is more convenient to compare two populations by using a **single overall rate** than it is by using a **set of many specific** rates. Interpretations can become difficult when the number of specific rates is large. Also, a single rate is especially convenient when additional variables of interest need to be brought into analysis at a later stage.

Nevertheless, you should also be able to perceive situations when an overall rate would be of questionable value. There are two situations that you can clearly recognize:

1. **If the comparison of interest is restricted to a subgroup that is still broadly defined,** then a confounding variable (e.g. age) may remain and you will need to adjust your rates. Moreover, a rate for the subgroup will be the focus, not an overall rate for the entire group.

2. **If there is a noticeable inconsistency in the direction of specific rates with respect to a confounding variable,** (i.e., specific rates are noticeably higher for one population at certain ages and/or noticeably lower at other ages), then no single overall rate for each population would highlight the age-specific differences. Use of an overall rate would tend to mask such differences, in this situation.

Problem 10:

Suppose you wished to compare two populations' mortality rates:

Table 3.1

	Population A	Population B
Young	12.2/1,000	10.3/1,000
Old	9.5/1,000	15.9/1,000

Would an overall rate be appropriate here?

Your Solution:

Problem 11:
What is the primary advantage of using an overall rate?

Your Solution:

Problem 12:
Can you give two reasons for **not** using overall rates?

Your Solution:

METHODS FOR RATE ADJUSTMENT

Returning to the dental epidemiologic research being conducted in Needlepoint Knoll and Textbooktown, we have determined that overall tooth mortality rates are of interest to us, but that the results are being biased because of the confounding factor, age. We would like to know what the overall tooth mortality rates would be in these two cities if the age structure of the population were the same in both locations. We can determine this mathematically by *adjusting* the rates that we have observed to conform to a *known standard population*.

Table 3.2

(1)	Needlepoint Knoll		Textbooktown		Standard	
	(2)	(3)	(4)	(5)	(6)	(7)
Age	Population	Rate	Population	Rate	Population	Rate
<35 years	23,000	1.0	40,000	3.0	30,000	2.0
35-65 years	45,000	2.0	25,000	5.0	33,000	5.2
>65 years	70,000	12.0	14,500	15.0	12,000	15.0
Total	**138,000**	**6.9**	**79,500**	**5.8**	**75,000**	**5.5**

If we utilize the "direct" method of adjustment, we will need the age-specific population distribution of the standard population, which appears in column 6 of Table 3.2, and the observed age-specific tooth mortality rates found in the two cities which appear in columns 3 and 5. If we utilize the "indirect" method of adjustment, we will need the age-specific tooth mortality rates of the standard population found in column 7, the observed age-specific population distribution of the two cities, listed in columns 2 and 4 and the overall tooth mortality rates i.e., 6.9 and 5.8. (Usually all the information presented in Table 3.2 is not available.)

DIRECT METHOD

To obtain the overall age adjusted tooth mortality rate for Needlepoint Knoll, by the *direct method,* each observed specific rate, 1.0, 2.0 and 12.0 is multiplied by the corresponding age specific standard population size. The sum of these three products is then divided by the total population of the standard.

$$[(1.0)(30,000) + (2.0)(33,000) + (12.0)(12,000)]/75,000 =$$
3.2 missing teeth per person

Problem 13:

What is the overall age adjusted tooth mortality rate for Textbooktown, Texas utilizing the direct method?

Your Solution:

As you can see, when we control for the confounding factor, age, the overall adjusted rates indicate the reverse of what is portrayed by the overall crude rates. If age was not a factor, Needlepoint Knoll with its optimum fluoride concentration would have a lower tooth mortality rate.

INDIRECT METHOD

In the *indirect method,* the concept is the same but the choice of weights is different. Instead of adjusting according to the standard age-specific **population size,** the standard age-specific **rates** are used to determine the rate of missing teeth that would be expected in our populations if the standard rates applied. This is done by multiplying the numbers found in columns 2 and 4 by the corresponding rate in column 7. The **observed** rate of missing teeth is divided by the **expected** rate that is calculated. The resulting ratio is called the standard tooth mortality ratio. If the event of interest were something other than tooth mortality, the name would be changed accordingly.

$$\frac{\text{Standard tooth}}{\text{mortality ratio}} = \frac{\text{Observed rate of missing teeth}}{\text{Expected rate of missing teeth}}$$

To obtain the overall adjusted rate, this standard mortality ratio is multiplied by the overall crude mortality in the standard population. For Needlepoint Knoll:

Expected rate of missing teeth =
$$[(23,000)(2.0) + (45,000)(5.2) + (70,000)(15.0)] / 138,000 =$$
1,330,000/138,000 = 9.64 missing teeth per person

Observed rate of missing teeth = 6.9

Standard tooth mortality ratio 6.9/9.64 = .72

Adjusted rate (.72)(5.5) = 3.96

Problem 14:

What is the overall age adjusted tooth mortality rate of Textbooktown, Texas, utilizing the indirect method?

Your Solution:

The numbers obtained by the direct and indirect methods differ, but the conclusions are the same. The actual results obtained will also vary depending on the standard that is selected. Adjustments are most commonly made for age, but can be made for any confounding factor, such as sex, income level, education level, etc., if the necessary information is available. The decision to use the direct or the indirect method is usually based on the type of stratum-specific data that are available. If the adjusted rates and the crude rates are equal, then the factor being adjusted for has no effect and is not creating a bias in the results.

REVIEW:

1) Overall rate: A summary statistic for a factor of interest for the total population.
2) Specific rate: The proportion with a factor of interest within a select stratum of the population.
3) Crude rate: A rate unadjusted for any confounding factors.
4) Adjusted rate: A rate adjusted for a confounding factor.
5) Direct adjusted rate: A rate adjusted by applying the stratum specific rates obtained from the data to a standard population.
6) Indirect adjusted rate: A rate adjusted by applying the stratum specific rates of a standard population to each stratum of the data set.
7) Both the overall and specific rates may be either crude or adjusted.

SOLUTIONS

Problem 1:

City B which has only .3 ppm of fluoride.

Problem 2:

age, fluoride concentration

Problem 3:

You are correct if you answered *confounding factor*.

Problem 4:

This question is a little tricky, so if you get it correct, you're either doing great or you took a lucky guess. The correct answer is *false* because the confounding factor *age* prevents *any* kind of reliable conclusion about the effect of fluoride using crude rates. If no difference in crude rates is observed, this too may be entirely due to difference in age structures between City A and City B. Similarly, any large difference might also be explained entirely by the age factor.

Problem 5:

confounding factor

Problem 6:

You are correct if you answered *yes* to all four questions, and wrote *tooth mortality rates for City A and City B, missing teeth* and *age* in the blanks for a, b, and d respectively.

Problem 7:

The answer is *No* because 1) you would not be interested in comparing overall rates, and 2) because age would not be a confounding factor.

Problem 8:

You are correct if you answered *specific*. You would be incorrect if you answered *overall*.

Problem 9:

overall

Problem 10:

The answer here should be *No* since the comparison of rates within age specific groups (broadly classified into old and young) differs greatly and the direction of the difference is not consistent.

Problem 11:

As a convenient summary index.

Problem 12:

You should have written something like:
1) the comparison is restricted to a specific age group, and
2) there is a noticeable inconsistency in the direction of age specific rates with respect to a confounding variable.

Problem 13:

$[(3.0)(30,000) + (5.0)(33,000) + (15.0)(12,000)]/75,000 = 5.8$ missing teeth per person

Problem 14:

$[(40.000)(2.0) + (25,000)(5.2) + (14,500(15.0)]/79,500 = 5.38$

Standard tooth mortality ratio $5.8/5.38 = 1.08$

Adjusted rate $(1.08)(5.5) = 5.94$

For further study see Colton, T., Statistics in Medicine, Boston, MA, Little Brown and Co. 1974, p. 47-51.

POSTTEST 3

Suppose you are a state dental director with a limited budget for dental programs. You want to find out which parts of the state are in greatest need of dental services. A survey is conducted at selected schools around the state to determine the oral health status of children in different communities. In some of the larger cities, the schools are located in neighborhoods that have differing socioeconomic status (SES). From your knowledge of dental epidemiology, you know that the factors that determine SES classification, such as income and education, are inversely related to the DMFT rate (number of decayed, missing and filled teeth per person) for a population. The data for children in two cities are as follows:

CITY A				CITY B		
SES	Population	DMFT Rate		SES	Population	DMFT Rate
High	5,000	1.5		High	20,000	1.7
Middle	30,000	1.8		Middle	40,000	2.1
Low	25,000	5.2		Low	10,000	7.3
Total	**60,000**	**3.2**		**Total**	**70,000**	**2.7**

Let's see if you can evaluate whether or not rate adjustment is appropriate for the data.

1) What are the four conditions for rate adjustment?
2) What is the confounding factor in this example?
3) Is the use of an overall rate appropriate?
4) How many of the four conditions for rate adjustment are satisfied?
5) Suppose the DMFT rate for low SES in City B was 4.1 instead of 7.3. Should you use rate adjustment?
6) If you think that rate adjustment is warranted to compare the DMFT rates for City A and City B, consider the standard population, City C.

CITY C		
SES	Population	DMFT Rate
High	10,000	1.6
Middle	35,000	2.0
Low	15,000	6.0
Total	**60,000**	**2.9**

Calculate the adjusted rates using the direct method. Calculate the adjusted rates using the indirect method.

YOUR ANSWERS TO POSTTEST 3

Name:

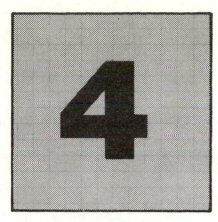

CHAPTER 4

FREQUENCY DISTRIBUTIONS

INTRODUCTION

When presented with a set of raw data, such as in Table 4.1 below, the reader can usually get only a vague impression from glancing over or "eye balling" the data. This is especially true when shown a large data set. Some form of visual simplification is essential for clearer understanding, and in this chapter we will consider several techniques for displaying data. These techniques include the frequency table, the histogram (or bar chart), the frequency polygon, and the cumulative frequency distribution.

Table 4.1

AGE AT TIME OF EMERGENCE OF MAXILLARY FIRST PREMOLARS (in years)					
10.5	10.7	9.5	10.5	11.8	9.7
12.0	10.3	13.5	12.3	10.6	11.2
10.7	11.5	11.1	10.6	9.3	9.8
10.4	7.5	10.2	8.7	10.9	12.9
11.7	10.3	10.6	10.5	11.9	9.9
13.9	10.6	10.0	10.8	10.6	11.0
7.3	8.0	8.5	12.5		

OBJECTIVES

You will be able to construct from a suitable set of raw data the following tables and charts:
1) frequency table
2) histogram
3) frequency polygon
4) cumulative frequency distribution.

FREQUENCY TABLE

Suppose the American Dental Association did a survey of dentists to determine the number of hours they worked per week. A sample of the results might look as follows:

5	10	33	22	21
35	38	40	55	41
45	31	45	40	33
32	35	20	24	34
37	25	50	30	40

10	27	22	50	28
36	36	51	35	35
32	18	35	40	38
15	27	31	35	48
40	38	48	37	20

The first thing that you might want to do before analyzing the data is to rearrange it into a logical sequence. Below, the data are arranged in ascending order. This new arrangement of data is called an **array.**

5	24	32	36	40
10	25	33	36	41
10	27	33	37	41
15	27	34	37	45
18	28	35	38	45
20	30	35	38	48
20	30	35	38	48
21	31	35	40	50
22	31	35	40	50
22	32	35	40	55

One way of summarizing these measurements is by using a **frequency table** as shown below:

Table 4.2

FREQUENCY TABLE OF NUMBER OF HOURS WORKED PER WEEK AS REPORTED BY DENTISTS

Hours worked per week	Frequency
1-10	3
11-20	4
21-30	10
31-40	24
41-50	8
51-60	1
Total	**50**

Appropriate class intervals for number of hours worked are chosen (1-10, 11-20, 21-30, 31-40, 41-50, 51-60) and the number of measurements falling within each class interval computed. In this case the class intervals are of equal width. This is often desirable but not necessary.

An important decision to be made when constructing frequency tables is the width of each class interval, since this will determine the number of intervals and hence the amount of detail with which the data will be reported.

About 5-10 class intervals are appropriate for most purposes. If there are less than 5 intervals too much information may be lost. More than 10 intervals may give too much detail and we lose our ability to obtain an overall feel for the distribution. Also, the total number of measurements will to some extent determine the number of intervals. It is inappropriate to have several intervals, each with just one or two measurements or to have a few intervals, each with large numbers of measurements. In many cases, intervals are chosen according to precedence. If other investigators have reported findings with certain intervals it may be desirable to use the same intervals so as to allow the data to be compared easily.

Problem 1:

Construct a frequency table from the data in Table 4.1 which lists the age of 40 children at the time of each maxillary first premolar eruption.

Your Solution:

RELATIVE FREQUENCY DISTRIBUTION

A relative frequency distribution is obtained by dividing the actual frequencies by the total number of observations and then multiplying by 100 to convert to a percentage. Note that the relative frequencies should add to approximately 100% (allow for rounding errors). This provides a check on the arithmetic. The relative frequency distribution for the frequency table shown in Table 4.2, "Number of Hours Worked per Week as Reported by Dentists" is presented below in Table 4.3.

Table 4.3

RELATIVE FREQUENCY DISTRIBUTION OF NUMBER OF HOURS WORKED PER WEEK AS REPORTED BY DENTISTS

Hours worked per week	Frequency	Relative frequency (%)
1-10	3	6
11-20	4	8
21-30	10	20
31-40	24	48
41-50	8	16
51-60	1	2
Total	**50**	**100**

Problem 2:
Determine the relative frequency distribution for the frequency table that you designed in Problem 1 which describes the age of children at the time of first maxillary premolar eruption.

Your Solution:

HISTOGRAM

A histogram or bar chart may be constructed from a relative frequency distribution by drawing a bar for each class interval corresponding to the relative frequency of occurrence of measurements in that interval. A histogram for the relative frequency of number of hours worked in Table 4.3 may be constructed as follows:

Figure 4.1

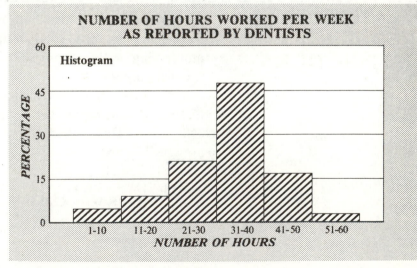

In a bar chart, the bars or columns are of equal width and there are spaces between the categories that the bars represent. The bars may be vertical or horizontal. Bar charts are excellent for visualizing comparisons among sets of data; chart is provided in Figure 4.2.

Figure 4.2

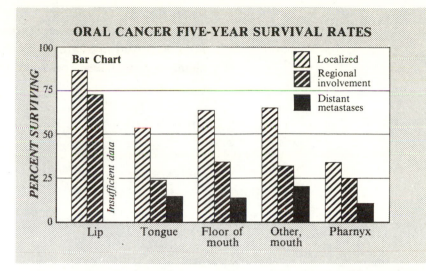

Although at first glance, histograms and bar charts may look very similar, histograms must be constructed much more cautiously. There is no space between the cells or bars, and the **area** enclosed by the bar (determined by multiplying its height times its width) represents the frequency distribution of the data. This will become more apparent in chapter 8. When the intervals represent an equal number of units, histograms are easy to construct. However, adjustments are necessary if the intervals are not equal (i.e. - they represent different numbers of days or hours) so that the areas outlined remain proportionate.

FREQUENCY POLYGON

A **frequency polygon** is often used in place of a histogram. Instead of constructing a bar over each class interval, a **dot is marked at the same height over the midpoint of the class interval.** These dots are **joined together by straight lines** to form a frequency polygon as shown in Figure 4.3. Many charts are constructed using this principle of displaying data.

Figure 4.3

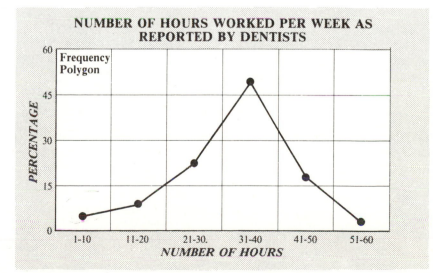

Problem 3:

Using the relative frequency distribution of "Age of Children at Time of Eruption of Maxillary First Premolar" that you determined in the last problem, construct both a histogram and a frequency polygon.

Your Solution:

CUMULATIVE FREQUENCY DISTRIBUTION

Finally, a **cumulative frequency distribution** may be constructed by calculating the **percentage of measurements below the upper limit for each class interval.** Returning to our example of number of hours worked by dentists, the cumulative distribution may easily be constructed using the relative frequency distribution in Table 4.3. In Table 4.4 below we see that 14% of the dentists reported working 20 or fewer hours a week. It is common to show relative and cumulative frequencies in the same table.

Table 4.4

RELATIVE AND CUMULATIVE FREQUENCY DISTRIBUTION OF NUMBER OF HOURS WORKED PER WEEK AS REPORTED BY DENTISTS

Hours worked per week	Frequency	Relative frequency (%)	Cumulative frequency (%)
1-10	3	6	6
11-20	4	8	14
21-30	6	12	26
31-40	28	56	82
41-50	8	16	98
51-60	1	2	100
Total	**50**	**100**	

Note: In some cases the total may not add up to exactly 100% because of errors caused by rounding to the nearest percentage.

REVIEW

1) Remember a frequency table is a specification of the number of measurements falling within each class interval. You have to define the class intervals. From 5 to 10 class intervals are appropriate for most frequency tables.

2) A relative frequency distribution is a specification of the number of measurements falling within each class interval divided by the total number of observations, then multiplied by 100 to convert to a percentage.

3) A histogram is constructed from a relative frequency distribution by drawing a bar for each class interval whose area corresponds to the relative frequency of occurrence of measurements in that interval.

4) A frequency polygon is a chart that is formed by placing a dot over the mid-point of the class interval corresponding to the relative frequency of occurrence of measurements in that interval. Then the points are joined by straight lines.

5) A cumulative frequency distribution table is constructed by calculating the percentage of measurements below the upper limit for each class interval.

SOLUTIONS

Problem 1:

The data are in ascending order in Table 4.5 If you arrayed your data in this manner you probably found it easier to work with. However, it is not necessary. The array shows that the data range from 7.3 to 13.9. Class intervals of length one year and starting at 7.00 are appropriate and a solution showing a frequency table is shown in Table 4.6. You may have chosen different class intervals, but if you obtained a similar table you did fine.

Table 4.5

AGE AT TIME OF EMERGENCE OF MAXILLARY FIRST PREMOLARS (IN YEARS)

7.3	9.7	10.4	10.6	11.1	12.0
7.5	9.8	10.5	10.6	11.2	12.3
8.0	9.9	10.5	10.7	11.5	12.5
8.5	10.0	10.5	10.7	11.7	12.9
8.7	10.2	10.6	10.8	11.8	13.5
9.3	10.3	10.6	10.9	11.9	13.9
9.5	10.3	10.6	11.0		

Table 4.6

A FREQUENCY TABLE FOR AGE AT TIME OF ERUPTION OF MAXILLARY FIRST PREMOLARS

Age Interval	Frequency
7.0- 7.9	2
8.0- 8.9	3
9.0- 9.9	5
10.0-10.9	17
11.0-11.9	7
12.0-12.9	4
13.0-13.9	2
Total	**40**

Table 4.7

Problem 2:

FREQUENCY DISTRIBUTION OF FIRST MAXILLARY PREMOLAR ERUPTION BY AGE

Age Interval	Frequency	Relative frequency (%)
7.0- 7.9	2	5.0
8.0- 8.9	3	7.5
9.0- 9.9	5	12.5
10.0-10.9	17	42.5
11.0-11.9	7	17.5
12.0-12.9	4	10.0
13.0-13.9	2	5.0
Total	40	100.0

Problem 3:

Figure 4.4

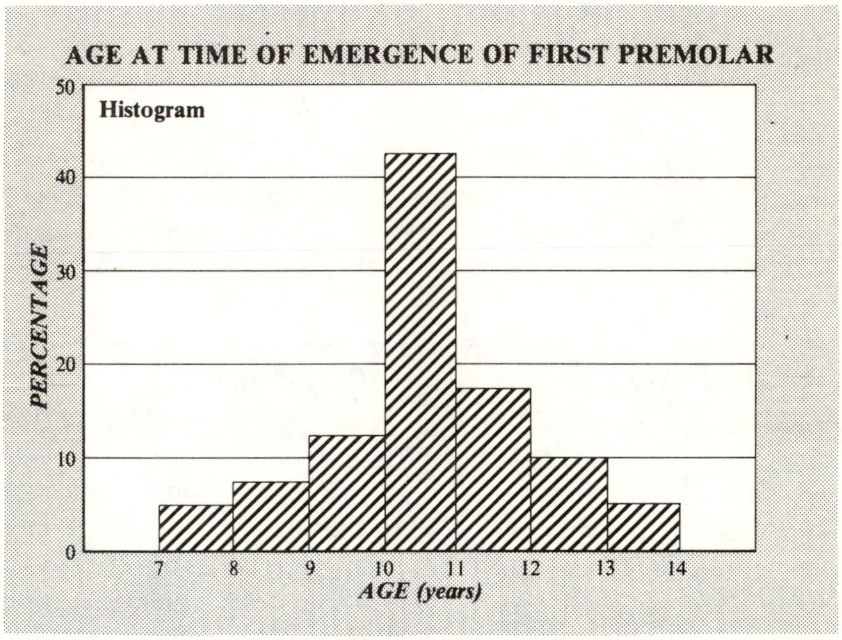

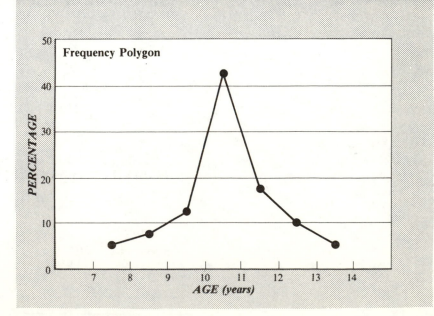

Figure 4.5

POSTTEST 4

1) First, look at the confusing unarrayed numbers in Table 4.8. These are the answers that were given by 25 people standing in line at the supermarket to the question, "When was your last visit to the dentist?"
2) Second, look at the same data, in arrayed form (Table 4.9).
3) Construct a frequency table, correctly labeling it "Length of Time Since Last Visit to the Dentist."
4) Next, calculate and add to the table the relative frequency and the cumulative frequency distributions.
5) Using the information in the Table 4.9, construct a bar chart.

Table 4.8

LENGTH OF TIME SINCE LAST VISIT TO THE DENTIST:
Unarrayed Raw Data

9 months	4 months	11 months
1 year	2 years 5 months	1 year 2 months
9 months	5 years	never
6 years	8 months	8 months
1 year 9 months	10 months	8 months
1 month	1 year 6 months	1 year 5 months
5 months	2 months	1 year 8 months
2 years	6 months	11 months
3 years 1 month		

Table 4.9

LENGTH OF TIME SINCE LAST VISIT TO THE DENTIST
Arrayed Raw Data

1 month	9 months	1 year 8 months
2 months	10 months	1 year 9 months
4 months	11 months	2 years
5 months	11 months	2 years 5 months
6 months	1 year	3 years 1 month
8 months	1 year 2 months	5 years
8 months	1 year 5 months	6 years
8 months	1 year 6 months	never
9 months		

YOUR ANSWERS
TO POSTTEST 4

Name:

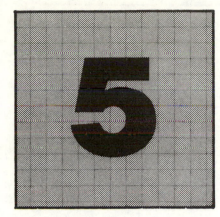

CHAPTER 5

MEASURES OF CENTRAL TENDENCY AND SPREAD

INTRODUCTION

It is important for dental and dental hygiene students to be able to understand the meaning of simple descriptive statistics since they are used commonly in professional journals and classroom lectures. In particular, in your clinical rotations and practicing career you will need to know something about descriptive statistics in making informed treatment decisions regarding pharmaceuticals, treatment methods, and surgical instruments. Also, you may need to calculate means and standard deviations of samples of data during some of your course work or for the research in which you are engaged during your dental education.

Dental care providers make measurements of patient attributes and form mental comparisons with a norm (or mean) to assist diagnosis. Sometimes there is consideration of how much spread or variation there is in the data. Standard deviation is a measure of spread and, like a mean, is a descriptive statistic.

This chapter is designed to explain **two types of descriptive statistics:** those which are average, or **measures of central tendency** such as mean and those which are **measures of spread** such as standard deviation.

OBJECTIVE

1) You will be able to calculate the **mean, median, mode, variance, range and standard deviation** of a given sample of data.

2) Given the following statements:

   a) *Half of all dentists practice more than 38 hours per week.*
   b) *On the average it takes 17 minutes to perform a class II cavity preparation on a bicuspid.*
   c) *More dentists practice with three operatories, two assistants, and a half-time hygienist than any other office staffing pattern.*

   you will be able to distinguish between what these statements say and what they *do not* say about the underlying populations in question.

CENTRAL TENDENCY

Measures of central tendency attempt to provide one sample statistic that describes the character of an entire data set. These statistics are *averages* and there are three of them - mean, mode and median.

The sample **mean** of a set of data items is the **arithmetic average.** To calculate the mean, add the items in the data set and divide by the number of items.

Problem 1:

Now, what is an appropriate synonym for the term *mean*?

Your Solution:

Now, suppose during one week an endodontist saw five patients who required therapy on their maxillary lateral incisor. Since an endodontic restoration must precisely fit the length of the root canal, knowledge of the mean length of teeth provides a starting point for this procedure. But ultimately the exact length of each tooth being treated must be known. Therefore, the endodontist measured the length of each tooth on the radiograph and found the measurements to be 19, 20, 21, 18 and 22 mm. The average length would be (19 + 20 + 21 + 18 + 22)/5 or 20 mm. By substituting symbols for these numbers we can develop a formula for calculating the mean of a sample. Think of the symbols x_1, x_2 . . ., etc. to x_n standing for individual items of a data set, where n is the total number of items. The sample mean, represented by the symbol $\bar{x}$ (pronounced "x-bar"), is calculated by the formula:

$$\bar{x} = \frac{x_1 + x_2 + \ldots + x_n}{n}$$

The symbol is commonly used in statistics to represent a sample mean.

You may be familiar with the "Σ" notation, pronounced "sigma," where Σ denotes **the sum of** all the x's, i.e., $x_1 + x_2 + \ldots + x_n$. Σ is merely a convenient shorthand notation. Using this notation the above expression may be written as:

$$\bar{x} = \frac{\Sigma x}{n}$$

Problem 2:

Suppose you measured the lengths of seven maxillary central incisors that were in need of endodontic treatment. The lengths were 21, 23, 29, 20, 18, 22 and 21 mm. What is the mean length of this sample of incisors?

Your Solution:

So the mean is easy to calculate. It is an average, or more technically, a measure of **central tendency** or **central location** in a set of data items. If we were told that the mean weight of a sample of seven men was 280 pounds we would get the impression we were dealing with a group of big men!

Median is another measure of central tendency. The sample median is the **middle item of a data set.** If data are arranged in order of increasing size, then the median will divide the data into two smaller but equal sized data sets. Half of the items are above the median, and half are below the median.

Problem 3:

Now try to think of the meaning of the term "median" without referring back to the previous sentences and write it below.

Your Solution:

In order to calculate the median of a sample of data, arrange the data in order of increasing size and then select the item in the middle. Sometimes there is a problem because with an even number of items in the data set there are two in the middle. In this case take the mean of these two items or scores. With an odd number there is no problem as there can only be one in the middle.

Problem 4:

Try calculating some medians. What is the median length of the 7 maxillary central incisors in the last exercise whose lengths were 21, 23, 29, 20, 18, 22, 21 mm?

Your Solution:

Problem 5:

Suppose now there was another patient whose maxillary central incisor was 25 mm long and his tooth is included to make a group of eight. What is the median length of these eight teeth?

Your Solution:

The **mode** is a third measure of central tendency that is often used to describe a data set. The mode is the **most frequently occurring item(s) in a set of data.** The mode may not be unique as **it is possible to have several modes in a data set.** For example, suppose 10 group practices were asked how many dental hygienists they employed and the replies were 0, 1, 1, 1, 2, 2, 3, 3, 3, 4 hygienists. There are two modes for this data set; there is a mode score at 1 and another at 3.

Problem 6:

Suppose another 10 group practices were asked the question, and the answers were as follows: 1, 5, 3, 6, 2, 1, 2, 5, 4, 3 dental hygienists. What is the mode(s) for this data set?

Your Solution:

You may wonder about the relative advantages of using mean, median, and mode as measures of central tendency or central location in a data set. Under most circumstances the mean is preferred. However, it has the disadvantage that it is influenced by extreme items in the data set. For instance, if one of the lateral incisors in the first example had been malformed and only 10 mm in length, the sample mean could have been 3 mm less. An extreme value has less influence on the sample median because the value of every item is not used up in computing the middle score. Thus, a high score does not pull the median up. The mode is generally a poor measure of central tendency since it may occur at an extreme value which gives no indication of where the data set is located. But a mode can provide an impression of the most frequent, or "popular," scores in a distribution. Surgical supply and drug salesmen often find modal statistics of dental practices and dentists' treatment patterns useful.

Problem 7:

Suppose you surveyed the patients sitting in the waiting rooms of several dental offices in a community and asked them how long they had to wait for a nonemergency appointment. The responses were as follows: 12, 3, 5, 2, 21, 8, 4, 7, 14, 3, 23 and 34 days. Calculate the sample mean, median and mode of this data set.

Which measure of central tendency would you use to describe the central tendency or location of this data set?

Your Solution:

SPREAD

Each of the 3 measures of central tendency can give important information about the data set. However, a summary in the form of central tendency alone is of limited value since it tells nothing about the amount of variability among the scores themselves. The following example illustrates this point.

After graduation from school, as you try to decide on a practice location, you may find it interesting to look at a table of statistics that tells you the mean net income of dental care providers located in different communities. If you have already decided that you want to practice in your hometown of 10,000 and see that the mean income of the seven dentists there is listed as $38,000/year you may be reluctant to return. You then learn, however, that this mean is greatly affected by two dentists who are nearly retired and practice only 2 or 3 half days per week. Upon inquiring about the range of incomes you learn that they range from $18,000 to $96,000. With this information you have a different impression of the activity within the dental practices in this community.

The range of a set of data is the highest item minus the lowest item. For the seven income values in this data set the range is enormous, which provides information on which to base a cautious interpretation of the mean statistic that you were originally given. Usually, information about the spread is as important as information about the central tendency of a data set. Range is one measure of spread.

Problem 8:
The systolic blood pressure measured for nine obese men was found to be 181, 175, 160, 182, 148, 180, 173, 175, and 192 mm Hg. What is the range of blood pressure for these men?

Your Solution:

The second measure of spread is **variance.** The larger the variance the more the data items are spread about the mean value. A variance of zero indicates no spread at all, i.e., all the scores have the same value. Sample variance is defined as **the sum of the squares of the deviations about the sample mean divided by one less than the total number of items.** A deviation about the sample mean is simply the difference between a data item and the mean of the data set. Using mathematical notation, the expression for variance may be written as,

$$s^2 = \frac{(x_1 - \bar{x})^2 + (x_2 - \bar{x})^2 + \ldots + (x_n - \bar{x})^2}{n-1}$$

where s^2 represents the sample variance of the data item, the x's, x_1, $x_2 \ldots x_n$, the individual data items, $\bar{x}$, the sample mean of the data items and n stands for the total number of data items.

Using the Σ notation, the same formula may be written as:

$$s^2 = \frac{\Sigma(x-\bar{x})^2}{n-1}$$

Note: The divisor is n-1, not n. The reason for this is theoretical and need not concern us here. (See page 55 for the Armitage reference.)

Problem 9:
Now write down the definition of variance in words without referring to the previous section.

Your Solution:

Problem 10:

You should now try a variance calculation. The atmospheric mercury vapor concentration was measured at five different locations in an office after an accidental spill occurred. The results were as follows: .01, .01, .03, .04, .06 mg Hg./m^3. What is the sample variance of these five mercury vapor levels?

Your Solution:

There is another way of writing the above variance formula which is often easier to apply, especially when using a desk calculator. The alternative formula is:

$$s^2 = \frac{x_1^2 + x_2^2 + \ldots + x_n^2 - \frac{1}{n}(x_1 + x_2 + \ldots + x_n)^2}{n-1}$$

or $$s^2 = \frac{(\text{sum of squares of data scores}) - \frac{1}{n}(\text{sum of data scores})^2}{n-1}$$

Using the Σ notation:

$$s^2 = \frac{\Sigma x^2 - \frac{1}{n}(\Sigma x)^2}{n-1}$$

Remember, Σx^2 is the sum of the squares of the data scores and $(\Sigma x)^2$ is the sum of the scores, squared.

Problem 11:

Now, repeat the calculation for the sample variance of the mercury vapor levels using the new formula.

Your Solution:

STANDARD DEVIATION

You should notice that the mean is measured in the same units as the data items but variance is measured in squared units. In order to overcome this, the square root of the variance is generally used as a measure of spread in preference to the variance itself. This quantity is known as the **standard deviation.**

s = sample standard deviation = $\sqrt{\text{sample variance}}$

The usual mathematical symbol for the standard deviation of a data set is s, but it is often notated as sd.

Problem 12:

What is the approximate standard deviation of the mercury vapor level in the above sample?

Your Solution:

One final point; some caution must be observed if **range** is used as a measure of spread, since it is **very much affected by extreme values.**

You should now be ready to take the Post Test. If there are any parts of this chapter you felt unsure about, read them over again. If you feel you have understood this presentation then try the post test. Good luck, but before you start, study the review.

REVIEW

1) Sample mean $= \overline{x} = \Sigma x / n$
2) Median $=$ middle data score
3) Mode(s) $=$ most frequently occurring data score(s)
4) Range $=$ (largest data score) - (smallest data score)

5) Sample variance $= \ s^2 = \dfrac{\Sigma(x-\overline{x})^2}{n-1} = \dfrac{\Sigma x^2 - \dfrac{1}{n}(\Sigma x)^2}{n-1}$

6) Sample standard deviation $= \sqrt{\text{sample variance}} = s.$

Problem 13:

Before taking the Post Test, try to identify the statistic referred to by each of the three statements which were listed just under the *Objective* on the first page of this chapter.

Your Solution:

SOLUTIONS

Problem 1:

If you wrote down *arithmetic average* you are doing fine. The concept of average is familiar to most people and a mean is the most commonly used average.

Problem 2:

22 mm. If you were not quite right, check your calculation. The total length of the seven teeth is 154 mm. If you divide 154 by 7 you get 22.

Problem 3:

If you wrote something like *the middle score in a data set* then you are on target.

Problem 4:

The answer is 21 mm. You should have arranged the lengths in increasing order and selected the middle item (i.e., 18, 20, 21, 21, 22, 23, 29). 21 is the middle item.

Problem 5:

The answer is 21.5 mm. However, you may have had some trouble here. If we arrange the lengths in increasing order we get 18, 20, 21, 21, 22, 23, 25, 29.

There are an even number of data items and the middle two are marked. The mean of these two is 21.5.

Problem 6:

If you rearranged the data scores in order you should have had no trouble. The scores rewritten in order are: 1, 1, 2, 2, 3, 3, 4, 5, 5, 6.

Four values occur twice and two values only once. All four that occur twice are the most frequently occurring and so there are four modes, i.e., at 1, 2, 3, and 5. So here is a data set for which the mode does not tell us very much about the central tendency in the distribution.

Problem 7:

If we arrange the waiting times in increasing order we have 2, 3, 3, 4, 5, 7, 8, 12, 14, 21, 23, 34.

For this data set there is a mode at 3, the mean is 11.3 and the median is 7.5. Here, the median is the most appropriate measure of central tendency since the 34 reading is an extreme value which has considerable influence on the mean. The mode at 3 is obviously not an appropriate measure of central location. It seems only to be a chance occurrence that there were two readings of 3.

Although the sample median is the appropriate measure of central tendency in this example, the sample mean is most commonly employed as an indicator of the central location. But always keep an eye out for extreme measures which are sometimes referred to as "outliers."

Problem 8:

The range is 44 mm Hg. In general, the surest way to proceed is to write down these blood pressures in increasing order of magnitude, checking off each item as you proceed:

148, 160, 173, 175, 175, 180, 181, 182, 192 mm Hg.
The range is 192 - 148 = 44 mm Hg.

If you took the short cut and scanned by eye, we hope you obtained the correct answer.

Problem 9:

Variance is a measure of the degree of spread of the data items. It is defined as the "sum of squares of deviations about the mean divided by the number of items minus one." This is the most difficult definition presented so far and so if you feel you have not grasped it yet, read the section over again.

Problem 10:

The answer is .00045 (mg Hg/m³)². If you were right you did well. If not, here is how to do the calculation. The formula we want to use is,

$$s^2 = \frac{\Sigma(x-\bar{x})^2}{n-1} = \frac{1}{n-1}\Sigma(x-\bar{x})^2$$

We first find

$$\bar{x} = \frac{\Sigma x}{n} = \frac{1}{5}(.01 + .01 + .03 + .04 + .06) = .03 \text{ mm Hg}/\text{m}^3$$

Then substituting the individual mercury vapor scores and in the formula for s^2, we get:

$s^2 = 1/5\text{-}1\ [(.01\text{-}.03)^2 + (.01\text{-}.03)^2 + (.03\text{-}.03)^2 + (.04\text{-} \qquad + (.06\text{-}.03)^2]$

$s^2 = 1/4\ [(-.02)^2 + (-.02)^2 + (0)^2 + (.01)^2 + (.03)^2]$

$s^2 = 1/4\ (.0004 + .0004 + 0 + .0001 + .0009)$

$s^2 = 1/4\ (.0018) = .00045\ (\text{mg Hg}/\text{m}^3)^2$

This completes the calculation.

Problem 11:

Did you get the same answer? You did? Good! The two formulas are, in fact, equivalent (this may be proved mathematically). The second formula is easier to use with a desk calculator as sums of squares are simple to compute whereas squares of differences are a bit more tedious. Also, if the data scores are whole numbers, the second has advantage over the first as that method may involve squaring decimals (as in the example you have just worked by the two methods).

Problem 12:

The answer is $\sqrt{.00045} \cong .02\ \text{mg Hg}/\text{m}^3$

Problem 13:

You should identify these statements as references to the 1) median, 2) mean, and 3) mode. Now try the Post Test.

See Armitage, P., Statistical Methods in Medical Research. Oxford, Boston. Blackwell Scientific Publications, 1971.

POSTTEST 5

A prosthodontist recorded the oral vertical dimension of ten new patients that required complete dentures. The measurements were: 7, 11, 10, 8, 5, 7, 9, 7, 6, 10 mm.

1) Calculate the mode(s), median and mean values of this sample of vertical dimension scores.
2) Determine the range in the vertical dimension scores recorded for these ten patients.
3) Calculate the sample variance and standard deviation of the vertical dimension scores for these patients.

YOUR ANSWERS TO POSTTEST 5

Name:

CHAPTER 6

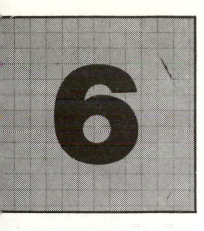

PROBABILITY

NTRODUCTION

"I have set my life upon a cast,
And I will stand the hazard of the die!"
Shakespeare, *Richard III*

The concept of probability plays an important role in patient care and scientific investigation because very few decisions regarding the prognosis of treatment or the results of research can be predicted with absolute certainty. One patient may want to know what his chances are of getting oral cancer. Another patient with oral cancer may want to know what his survival chances are for the next five years. However, it is difficult to think of probabilities in terms of the individual patient who is your immediate concern. It is necessary, therefore, to generalize a given patient's situation and view it as *one* of many observations that have occurred in the past of similar patients in similar circumstances.

But first, one needs to understand the basic mathematical rules that govern the area of probability.

OBJECTIVE

1. You will be able to define **probability** and compute simple probability values.
2. You will be able to use the **Addition Law of Probability** to determine the probability of either of two events occurring.
3. You will be able to use the **Multiplication Law of Probability** to determine the probability of both of two events' occurring.

ROBABILITY

Definition: Probability is a mathematical measure of the likelihood that an event will occur in repeated trials under similar conditions, and at a determinable frequency.

In 1977, there were 12,835 dental school applicants for 5,954 available places. Forty-six percent of the applicants were accepted. The outcome of each applicant can be considered a separate trial or event which in this case was repeated 12,835 times under similar conditions. The probability of event A where A is "an applicant

accepted to dental school in 1977" is .46. This is written in th
following notation:

$$P(A) = .46$$

and is read, "the probability of A is .46."

Probabilities may also be expressed as decimals, fractions o
percentages. If they are expressed as decimals or fractions, the possib
range of values is from 0 to 1. A probability of 0 indicates that it
impossible for an event to occur. A probability of 1 indicates tha
it is certain to occur. If expressed as a percentage, the range of valu
is from 0.00 to 100.00 percent.

When calculating probabilities, all possible outcomes of an ever
must be determined. The sum of the probabilities assigned to each o
the possible mutually exclusive outcomes must add up to 1. In th
above example, there are two possible outcomes: either a candida
is accepted or is not accepted, that is, either event A occurs or it do
not. These are called **complementary events.** Since the sum of thes
two probabilities must equal 1, the probability of not A, written a
$P(\overline{A})$ or $P(A)$, is as follows:

$$P(\overline{A}) = 1 - P(A)$$

Substituting .46 for P(A) we can determine that $P(\overline{A}) = 1 - .46 = .5$
These are called **mutually exclusive events** because either one or th
other will occur. They cannot both occur as the outcome of the san
trial. For each flip of a coin, the outcome is either heads or tai
(assuming that it is a fair coin). For each roll of a die, the outcome
either a 1, 2, 3, 4, 5, or 6. These are mutually exclusive events. If the
are "n" number of equally likely outcomes of an event, th
probability of each event occurring is $1/n$. For each roll of the d
there are six possible outcomes, all of which are equally likely. Th
probability of rolling a "3" is $1/6$ and is equal to P(rolling a 4)
P(rolling a 5), etc. The $P(1) + P(2) + P(3) + P(4) + P(5) + P(6) =$

Returning now to our dental school applicants who are a
nervously waiting for that fateful letter or telephone call. If the ou
comes are designated as successes or failures and there are N_s su
cesses and N_f failures, the total number of outcomes is $N_s + N_f$. I
this case, $N_s = 5,954$, for number of successes and the total numbe
of cases, both successes and failures is 12,835. The probability o
event A (success) can be calculated by:

$$P(A) = N_s/(N_s + N_f) = 5,954/12,835 = .46$$

(Note: We are assuming here that all the applicants were equal
qualified and had an equal chance of being selected. The winners
this professional lottery, certainly know this is not true!)

Problem 1:

In a certain dental school, 125 senior dental students took th
Northeast Regional Board Licensing Examination. 110 studen
passed the examination. What was the probability of passing th
examination? What was the probability of not passing th
examination?

Your Solution:

It is not always the case that each outcome has the same chance of occurring. In a given population:

P(Class I occlusion) = .70
P(Class II occlusion) = .25
P(Class III occlusion) = .05

These are the three possible types of occlusion and they are mutually exclusive. The sum of their probabilities is 1.

ADDITION RULE OF PROBABILITY

The probability that any one of two or more mutually exclusive events will occur is the sum of the probabilities of each event.

P(A or B) = P(A) + P(B)
P(A or B or C) = P(A) + P(B) + P(C),

where A, B and C are mutually exclusive.

The probability that a person selected at random from the above population has either a Class I or a Class II occlusion is expressed as:

P(Class I or Class II) = P(Class I) + P(Class II) =
.70 + .25 = .95

This happens to be the same as the probability of not having a Class III occlusion which would be expressed as:

1 - P(Class III) = 1 - .05 = .95

Problem 2:

In a certain neighborhood health center with 4,250 active patients, payments for dental services were either paid directly by the patient, by Medicaid or by a private insurance carrier. If there are 2,210 patients paying directly "out of pocket," and 510 patients have private dental insurance coverage, what is the probability that a patient will have some type of insurance, either Medicaid or private insurance?

Your Solution:

The situation becomes more complicated if the events are not mutually exclusive. If there is an overlap between two categories, they can be visualized in the following diagram by the two overlapping circles A and B. The shaded area in the center, C, could be considered as belonging to both A and B.

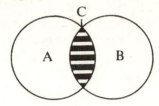

In a group of adults who have first molars that are decayed or filled, there may be some teeth that are both decayed and filled. Suppose:

15 teeth are decayed
80 teeth are filled
5 teeth are decayed and filled

We have:

P(any decay present) =
P(teeth decayed or decayed and filled) =
.15 + .05 = .20
P(any restoration present) =
P(teeth filled or decayed and filled) =
.80 + .05 = .85

As you can see, the "decayed and filled" group is being counted twice, and as a result the sum of the two probabilities do not equal one. Thus, if we were to consider the category, "any decay present" and the category, "any restoration present" as the only two possible outcomes in this example and assume that these are mutually exclusive events, we would get a probability greater than 1 and our assumption would be incorrect.

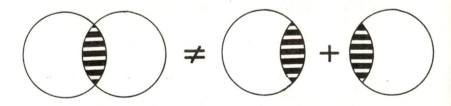

In the case where two events are not mutually exclusive, the following formula applies:

P(A or B) = P(A) + P(B) - P(A and B)

This is the general case of the addition rule of probability. If the two events A and B are mutually exclusive, then the probability of both A and B occurring is zero and the last term in the equation, P(A and B), can be ignored. Thus:

P(any decay present or any restoration present) =
P(any decay present) + P(any restoration present)
- P(any decay and restoration present)=
.20 + .85 - .05 = 1.00

Problem 3:

Another group of adults who have a caries free dentition is added to the sample. The first molars now under consideration fall into the following categories:

40 are sound

15 decayed

80 filled

5 decayed and filled

What is the probability of any first molar selected at random being only decayed? Having any decay? Being only "decayed and filled?" Having any filling? Having any decay or any filling?

Your Solution:

INDEPENDENT EVENTS AND THE MULTIPLICATION RULE

If the occurrence or non-occurrence of one event in no way affects the other, then these events are said to be independent. To determine the probability that two independent events, A and B, both occur, one need only multiply the probability of each individual event occurring. If A and B are independent, then:

$$P(A \text{ and } B) = P(A) \cdot P(B)$$

The concept of independent events is different from that of mutually exclusive events. Two events can be independent, but not mutually exclusive. For example, if two dice are tossed simultaneously, the outcome of *each* die is independent, that is, one toss in no way affects the other regardless of what numbers appear on each die.

Consider "A" as the outcome of the first die and "B" as the outcome of the second die and "C" as the sum of the two outcomes. If A=3 and B=3, then events A=3 and B=3 are independent but not mutually exclusive because rolling a "3" on one die does not exclude the possibility of rolling a "3" on the other.

If $A = 5$ and $C = 11$, then A and C are not independent because the result C depends on both A and B. If $B = 6$ and $C = 11$, then B and C are not mutually exclusive because both events can occur.

For any two independent events that are not mutually exclusive:

$$P(A \text{ or } B) = P(A) + P(B) - (P(A) \cdot P(B))$$

This is similar to the formula used on page 62 but now the last term P(A and B) can be substituted by P(A) · P(B).

In the above example of A=5 and B=6,

P(A or B) = (1/6) + (1/6) - ((1/6) · (1/6)) = 11/36

For many genetic diseases, such as osteogenesis imperfecta, the probability that a given couple will have affected children is the same from one birth to another. That is, the probability of an affected child on one birth has no effect on the probability of affected children on subsequent births. For a given couple the probability of:

an affected son = 1/4

a normal son = 1/4

an affected daughter = 0

a normal daughter = 1/2

What is the probability of two affected sons on two successive births? Since each birth is an independent event,

P(affected son and affected son) =

P(affected son) · P(affected son) =

1/4 · 1/4 = 1/16

Problem 4:

For the couple mentioned above, what is the probability that they first have an affected son and then have a normal daughter? Again assume that the probability of an affected child at one birth has no effect on the probability of affected children in subsequent births.

Your Solution:

Unfortunately, events in life are not always independent and thus calculating the probability of their occurrence becomes more complex.

Suppose you knew that the probability of the mesial surface of the maxillary right lateral incisor becoming decayed was .20, and the probability of the distal surface of the maxillary right central incisor becoming decayed was .15. If you used the multiplication rule for independent events, you would expect that the probability of both the mesial and distal surfaces of these teeth being decayed would be .20 × .15 = .03. However, from clinical experience one knows that if the mesial surface of one tooth becomes decayed, it is more likely that the adjacent distal surface will also be decayed. The probability of both surfaces being decayed might be .13 rather than .03. An adjustment needs to be made in the formula to account for these types of circumstances.

CONDITIONAL PROBABILITIES

Quite often a certain event is more or less likely to occur if another event has already occurred. For example, if an individual has been smoking heavily for most of his life, he is more likely to have oral cancer than someone who has never smoked. A young child is more likely to develop rampant caries if all his older siblings who live at home have rampant caries than if they were all caries-free. When the probability of an event is altered or restricted because another event or condition has occurred, it is referred to as a **conditional probability** and is written *P(A/B)* and read "the probability of A *given* that B has occurred."

The general form of the multiplication rule which can be used when events are not independent, but one is dependent or conditional upon the other is:

　　1) P(A and B) = P(B/A) P(A) = P(A/B) P(B).

When events A and B are independent, then

　　2) P(A/B) = P(A) and

　　3) P(B/A) = P(B)

because the probability of A will be the same regardless of whether or not B has occurred.

Substituting line 3 into equation 1, one gets

$$P(A \text{ and } B) = P(B) \cdot P(A)$$

which is equivalent to the previous formula that was used.

Suppose on a Friday night, you are taking a short break from studying and decide to play a game of cards with your friends. What is the probability that on two successive draws, without replacing the cards, from a deck of cards we will draw a seven and then an eight? Remember that P(8/7) is read: 'Probability of drawing an 8 given that a 7 has already been drawn.

Your solution would be:

$$P(7 \text{ and } 8) = P(7) \cdot P(8/7)$$
$$P(7 \text{ on 1st draw}) = 4/52$$

P(8/7) = P(8) given that we have already drawn a seven. Since we draw without replacing, then if we drew a seven first, that would leave 51 cards of which 4 would be eight. Thus P(8/7) = 4/51 and

$$P(7 \text{ and } 8) = (4/52)(4/51) = (1/13)(4/51) = 4/663$$

Problem 5:

What is the probability that you draw a 7 and then another 7 on two successive draws from a 52 card deck without replacing the first card before drawing the second?

Your Solution:

REVIEW

1) **Addition Rule of Probability,** the "OR" rule general form:

$$P(A \text{ or } B) = P(A) + P(B) - P(A \text{ and } B)$$

For mutually exclusive events: $P(A \text{ or } B) = P(A) + P(B)$

For independent but not mutually exclusive events:

$$P(A \text{ or } B) = P(A) + P(B) - [P(A) \cdot P(B)]$$

2) **Multiplication Rule of Probability,** the AND rule general form:

$$P(A \text{ and } B) = P(B/A) \, P(A)$$

Independent events:

$$P(A \text{ and } B) = P(A) \cdot P(B)$$

$$P(B/A) = P(B)$$

SOLUTIONS

Problem 1:

P(Passing the Exam) = 110/125 = .88

P(Not Passing the Exam) = 1−.88 = .12

Problem 2:

P(Direct Payment) = 2210/4250 = .52

P(Private Insurance) = 510/4250 = .12

P(Direct) + P(P.I.) + P (Medicaid) = 1.0

P(Medicaid) = 1.0 - (.52 + .12)

P(Medicaid) = .36

P(Medicaid or P.I.) = P(Medicaid) + P(P.I.) = .36 + .12 = .48

Equivalently, P(Medicaid or P.I.) = 1 - P(Direct) = 1 - .52 = .48

Problem 3:

P(only decayed) = 15/140 = .11

P(any decay) = 15/140 + 5/140 = 20/140 = .14

P(only "decayed and filled") = 5/140 = .04

P(any filling) = 80/140 + 5/140 = 85/140 = .61

P(any decay or any filling) = 20/140 + 85/140 - 5/140 = 100/140 = .71

Problem 4:

The correct answer is 1/8. Using the multiplication theorem,
P(affected son and normal daughter) = P(affected son)
· P(normal daugher) = (1/4)(1/2) = 1/8

Problem 5:

The correct answer is 1/221.
The P(7 and 7) = P(7) · P(7/7 on first draw)
P(7 on first draw) = 4/52
P(7/7) = 3/51 since given you drew a seven on the first draw there
would be only 3 sevens remaining among 51 cards.
Therefore: P(7 and 7) = 4/52 · 3/51 = 3/663 = 1/221

POSTTEST 6

A young woman, Jenny, has recently moved to Boston from North Carolina and is having difficulty choosing from among the many modes of dental care delivery that are available to her. She is concerned with cost, quality and convenience and decides to investigate the dental school clinic. When she stops by to make an appointment she learns that she can be treated by beginning dental students, senior dental students, or faculty. (What she really wants is a prophylaxis from a dental hygienist.) Depending on who renders the necessary service, the time and cost will vary.

Table 6.1

TIME TO COMPLETE 2 SURFACE RESTORATION		
Type of practitioner	No.	Hours
Beginning students	96	3.0
Senior students	90	1.5
Faculty	14	.2

a) If Jenny is randomly assigned to a practitioner, what is the probability that she will be assigned to a faculty member?
b) If her sister, Susan, decides to make an appointment, what is the probability that she will be assigned to a senior student?
c) What is the probability of Jenny and Susan both being assigned to a beginning student assuming that it is possible for the same student to treat both of them?
d) What is the probability that Jenny or Susan will be assigned to a beginning student?
e) What is the probability of Jenny and Susan both being assigned to a beginning student assuming that the school has a rule that forbids the same dental student to treat siblings?
f) In which case(s), sections c, d or e, are the two events independent?

YOUR ANSWERS TO POSTTEST 6

Name:

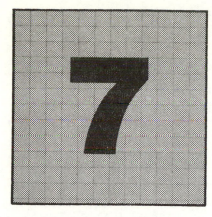

CHAPTER 7

EMPIRIC RISK AND THE BINOMIAL

INTRODUCTION

After working the first chapter dealing with probability, you should be familiar with one way of defining probability and with the additive and multiplicative rules for computing certain probabilities (e.g., P(A or B) and P(A and B)). In this chapter we introduce another, more general, probability definition and discuss what is meant by empiric risk. We will present another rule for calculating certain probabilities.

OBJECTIVE

1) You will be able to define the probability of an event in terms of the relative frequency with which that event has occurred in the past.
2) You will be able to estimate the empiric risk of an event by using the probability of that event as determined by the relative frequency definition.
3) You will be able to calculate the probability that a given event will occur exactly r times out of n independent identical trials when the probability that it will occur on a single trial is p.

PROBABILITY DEFINITION

In the last chapter we determined the probability of one event "A," occurring in an experiment that has n equally likely separate outcomes as $1/n$. If the event can occur more than once or more than one way, the probability of A is the ratio of the number of ways in which A can occur to the total number of possible outcomes or A/n. For example, if a pair of dice are tossed, there are 36 possible outcomes for the pair of numbers appearing on the top of the die. However, there are four ways that the event A, "sum equal to 5," can occur (1 and 4, 4 and 1, 2 and 3, 3 and 2). Thus P(sum of 5) = 4/36 = .11. Although this is an adequate definition it is not broad enough to cover the many situations in which n equally likely separate outcomes do not exist or we have no way of knowing what they are.

A second broader definition of probability is based on the fact that if a particular situation or experiment is repeated an indefinite number of times then the relative frequency of the occurrence of a particular outcome, A, tends to converge to a constant value which we call the probability of A.

$$P(A) = a/n$$

where a = number of times A occurred

and n = total number of trials

For any finite sequence of trials of an experiment, the observed relative frequency, a/n, of A is an **estimate** of the probability of A. If the number of trials is large, we can reasonably expect that the observed relative frequency will be close to the theoretical relative frequency or **true probability** of A. However, do not forget that we will never really know the true probability of A. We can only estimate it empirically, that is, by observation.

Problem 1:

You wish to know the probability of getting "heads" when you flip a coin. So you flip the coin ten times and find that heads comes up 4 times. Based on this experiment what is the probability of getting heads on a single toss?

Your Solution:

Problem 2:

You repeat the above 4 more times and obtain the following results:

Table 7.1

RESULTS			
Trial	No. Flips	No. Heads	Rel. Freq.
First	10	4	.4
Second	10	6	_____
Third	10	5	_____
Fourth	10	4	_____
Fifth	10	5	_____
Total	50	24	_____

Compute the relative frequency for each trial and the total.

Your Solution:

EMPIRIC RISK

The relative frequency approach to estimating probabilities is commonly used in clinical medicine because there may be no other way of determining the desired probabilities. This is a situation often encountered in genetic counseling and will serve to introduce you to the concept of empiric risk.

For many genetic diseases such as phenylketonuria (PKU), hemophilia A, and others, the mode of inheritance is known and the probability that a particular couple will have an affected child can be worked out on theoretical grounds. However, there are many other genetic diseases such as schizophrenia, cleft-lip and diabetes mellitus, in which the genetic mechanism is subject to debate. In order to determine probabilities in these cases we must resort to the relative frequency approach.

An **empiric risk** is a probability that is derived from the pooled data of many similar cases without regard to the genetic mechanism(s) of the hereditary trait involved. Specifically in this situation, it is the probability that children of an individual(s) affected with a hereditary disease will also be affected. Although empiric risk figures may be useful guides, you should keep in mind that they are only general averages based on many experiences and *do not* necessarily accurately estimate the risk in a specific family.

For example let us consider "cleft lip, with or without cleft palate," CL(P). This is a condition with a definite genetic component. At present the exact genetic mechanism is under debate. Indeed, the condition may well represent a heterogeneous collection of different genetic causes. In American whites it has an incidence at birth near 1/1000, whereas in blacks the figure is closer to 1/2500. If a patient has cleft lip and/or palate the following table gives some empiric risks that a particular child of the patient will be born with a cleft.

Table 7.2

CL(P) MOTHER'S RISK OF HAVING A CHILD WITH CL(P)		
Number of Mother's Affected Parents	Number of Mother's Affected Siblings	Empiric Risk of Child Being Affected
0	0	.001
0	1	.04
0	2	.09
1	0	.04
1	1	.20

Problem 3:

What is the empiric risk that a pregnant woman with CL(P) whose father and sister also had CL(P), but whose husband and all other relatives are unaffected, will have a child with CL(P)?

Your Solution:

BINOMIAL

The binomial formula, $(p + q)^n$, provides us with a means of determining the probability of observing a specific number of successes in n trials. For example, if the probability that a certain couple will have a child with PKU (phenylketonuria) on any given pregnancy is $1/4$, and if this couple plan to have four children, then what is the probability that they will have exactly:

1) four children with PKU (i.e., 0 unaffected children)?
2) three children with PKU (i.e., 1 unaffected child)?
3) two children with PKU (i.e., 2 unaffected children)?
4) one child with PKU (i.e., 3 unaffected children)?
5) zero children with PKU (i.e., 4 unaffected children)?

The binomial expansion can give us the answers to these questions.

$$p = \text{probability of occurrence on a single trial.}$$

If we consider PKU as the occurrence of this event, then $p = 1/4$.

q = probability of failure of occurrence on a single trial =

$$1-p= 3/4.$$

n = the total number of trials = 4 (i.e. four children)

The binomial expansion is:

$$(p+q)^n = (p+q)^4 = p^4 + 4p^3q^1 + 6p^2q^2 + 4p^1q^3 + q^4$$

$$p^4 = (1/4)^4 = 1/256 =$$
$$\text{p(exactly four children with PKU)} = .0039.$$

$$4p^3q^1 = 4(1/4)^3(3/4) = 12/256 =$$
$$\text{p(exactly three children with PKU)} = .0469.$$

$$6p^2q^2 = 6(1/4)^2(3/4)^2 = 54/256 =$$
$$\text{p(exactly two children with PKU)} = .2109.$$

$$4p^1q^3 = 4(1/4)(3/4)^3 = 108/256 =$$
$$\text{p(exactly one child with PKU)} = .4219.$$

$$q^4 = (3/4)^4 = 81/256 =$$
$$\text{p(exactly zero children with PKU)} = .3164.$$

Notice that the power to which p is raised indicates how many successes (in this case PKU children) and the power to which q is raised indicates the number of failures (in this case unaffected children). Also notice that the sum of all five probabilities equals 1.0 and that for any individual term of the expansion the sum of the exponents of p and q equals n, the number of trials.

Problem 4:

Given the following binomial expansions, answer the question below.

$$(p+q)^2 = p^2 + 2p^1q^1 + q^2$$
$$(p+q)^3 = p^3 + 3p^2q^1 + 3p^1q^2 + q^3$$
$$(p+q)^4 = p^4 + 4p^3q^1 + 6p^2q^2 + 4p^1q^3 + q^4$$
$$(p+q)^5 = p^5 + 5p^4q^1 + 10p^3q^2 + 10p^2q^3 + 5p^1q^4 + q^5$$

If a particular couple are to have a total of three children and the probability that they will have a child with a cleft lip and/or palate on any particular birth is 1/5, then what is the probability that none of their children will be affected?

Your Solution:

Problem 5:
If the couple in problem 4 are to have five children instead of 3 what is the probability that exactly four of them will have a cleft lip and/or palate?

Your Solution:

APPLYING THE MULTIPLICATION AND ADDITION RULES

Why does the binomial work? What is the origin of each of the terms of the expansion? The fact is that we do not really need the binomial to work out the probabilities; we can use the multiplication and addition rules that we learned in the previous chapter. Recall the multiplication rule:

$$P(A \text{ and } B) = P(A) \cdot P(B/A)$$

where $P(B/A) = P(B)$ for A and B independent.

This rule may be extended to the following:

$$P(A \text{ and } B \text{ and } C \text{ and } \ldots N) = P(A) \cdot P(B) \cdot P(C) \ldots P(N)$$

for A, B, C, ... N independent

Also recall the addition rule:

$$P(A \text{ or } B) = P(A) + P(B) - P(A \text{ and } B)$$

where $P(A \text{ and } B) = 0$ for mutually exclusive events

This rule can be extended:

$$P(A \text{ or } B \text{ or } C \text{ or } \ldots N) = P(A) + P(B) + P(C) + \ldots + P(N)$$

for A, B, C, ... N mutually exclusive

Since separate births can be considered **independent** and having one type of family is **mutually exclusive** of any other type, the extensions of these two rules may be applied.

For example, if we asked the question: "For a couple whose chance of having a child with agenesis of one or more teeth on any single birth is 1/4, what is the probability if they have three children that their *first* child will have hypodontia (HD) and the *last two* will not have this condition (N)?" We are asking for

P(1st HD and 2nd N and 3rd N) = P(HD) · P(N) · P(N) =

(1/4)(3/4)(3/4) = 9/64

Notice that if p is probability of HD on a single birth and q is 1-p that the above expression is simply:

$$p^1 q^2$$

In the above example the question was *not* what is the probability of one child with hypodontia. Instead it was: "What is the probability that only the *first* child will have HD?" In order to answer the question: "What is the probability that exactly one child has HD?", we have to consider the ways in which we can have a family of three with exactly one affected. This can occur in the following ways:

A) 1st HD and 2nd N and 3rd N = (1/4)(3/4)(3/4) = 9/64

B) 1st N and 2nd HD and 3rd N = (3/4)(1/4)(3/4) = 9/64

C) 1st N and 2nd N and 3rd HD = (3/4)(3/4)(1/4) = 9/64

The probability of A, B and C above is each $p^1 q^2$ or 9/64. The probability of exactly one child with HD = P(A or B or C) = P(A) + P(B) + P(C) since A, B and C are mutually exclusive. This is equal to $3p^1 q^2$ which is the term of the binomial expansion of $(p+q)^3$ which we would have used to answer the question.

Thus the exponential part of a particular term in the expansion is the probability that a particular order will occur and the coefficient is the number of different orders that give the same overall breakdown of successes to failures.

GENERAL TERM OF THE BINOMIAL

With the following formula we can compute any term of any binomial much more easily and quickly than by completely expanding the binomial.

The probability of *exactly* r successes out of n trials is given by

$$\frac{n!}{(n-r)!\ r!}\ p^r\ q^{(n-r)}$$

when the probability of a success on any single trial is p and the probability of failure (1-p) is q. The notation n! is read "n factorial" and is

$$n \cdot (n-1) \cdot (n-2) \cdot (n-3) \ldots 1$$

for example 5! = 5·4·3·2·1 = 120. We define 0! as being equal to 1. In addition you should remember that any number raised to the zero power is equal to 1 (i.e., X^0 = 1) and any number raised to the one power is equal to itself (i.e., X^1 = X). Remember

$$0! = 1$$
$$X^0 = 1$$
$$X^1 = X$$

Example: If a man with dentinogenesis imperfecta (a disorder resulting from an autosomal dominant gene) is married to a normal woman and they have five children, what is the probability that exactly zero of them will develop the disorder? In this family the probability that any single child received the dentinogenesis imperfecta gene from the father and will thus develop the disease is 1/2.

Answer:
p = p(success on a single trial, developing the disorder) = 1/2
q = 1-p = 1/2 = p(being normal)
n = number of trials = 5
r = number of successes (i.e., the number with the disease) = 0

$$\frac{n!}{(n-r)!\ r!}\ p^r\ q^{(n-r)} = \frac{5!}{(5-0)!\ 0!}\ p^0\ q^{(5-0)}$$

$$\frac{5\times4\times3\times2\times1}{(5\times4\times3\times2\times1)\,(1)}\ \left(\frac{1}{2}\right)^0 \left(\frac{1}{2}\right)^5 = 1\cdot1\cdot\left(\frac{1}{2}\right)^5 = \frac{1}{32}$$

Problem 6:

In the above family what is the probability that exactly one child out of the 5 will have this disorder?

Your Solution:

Problem 7:

Consider the PKU problem we discussed earlier: recall that the probability of PKU on a single birth is 1/4 and we determined that the probability of exactly one child with PKU out of four was 108/256. To obtain this answer we had n = 4, r = 1, p = p(PKU) = 1/4, q = 3/4. Now answer the same question (i.e., in this family of four children, what is the probability that exactly one child will have PKU?) only this time define a success as being a normal child.

Your Solution:

n =
r =
p = p(normal child) = 3/4
q =

Note: It does not matter how you define a success as long as you get the right number of successes to answer the question (i.e., if PKU is a success then you need 1 success out of 4 children to answer the question whereas if normal is a success then you need three successes out of 4 children to answer the same question).

Problem 8:

For a particular couple the probability that they will have a child with Amelogenesis Imperfecta is 1/4. This couple wants to have 3 children. What is the probability that they will have *at least* one child with this enamel disorder?

Your Solution:

SOLUTIONS

Problem 1:

The correct answer is .4 since the relative frequency of heads was 4/10.

Problem 2:

For the 2nd, 3rd, 4th and 5th trials you should have calculated relative frequencies of .6, .5, .4 and .5 respectively. The total is 24/50 or 0.48. Thus our *estimate* of the probability of heads on any single flip is .48. Intuitively you should realize that as the number of flips on which this estimate is based increases our estimate will get closer to the theoretical true probability of .5.

Problem 3:

The correct answer from Table 7.2 is .20. That is, in 20% of all such recorded situations in the past a child with CL(P) has been born. *Remember: This figure comes from pooled data without regard to the genetic mechanism in any particular family. This condition may be the result of an autosomal dominant gene for example, in which case the RISK of a child having CL(P) would be 50%.*

Problem 4:

Since there are to be three children, n=3, and we must use $(p+q)^3$. In this problem we may define p as being the probability of having a cleft lip and/or palate, thus p = 1/5. q = 1-p = 4/5. Since we have let p be the probability of being affected and the question asked for the probability of zero affected out of three, then we must use the term of the expansion in which p is raised to the zero power. This term is q^3, since $q^3 p^0 = q^3 \cdot 1 = q^3$ *(Recall that any number raised to the zero power equals 1.0)*. Therefore the answer is:

$$q^3 = (4/5)^3 = (4/5)(4/5)(4/5) = 64/125 \text{ or about } 1/2.$$

Problem 5:

Here n=5, p=1/5 = probability of being affected, q = 1-p = 4/5 and we must use the term of the binomial $(p+q)$ in which p is raised to the 4th power. Thus:

$$5p^4 q^1 = 5(1/5)^4(4/5)^1 = 5(1/5)(1/5)(1/5)(1/5)(4/5) = 4/625 \text{ or } < 1\%.$$

Problem 6:

If you got 5/32 for your answer then you are correct.
n=5, r=1, p=1/2, and q=1-p=1/2.

$$\frac{5!}{(5-1)!1!} \quad (1/2)^1(1/2)^{5-1} = \frac{(5 \cdot 4 \cdot 3 \cdot 2 \cdot 1)}{(4 \cdot 3 \cdot 2 \cdot 1)(1)} \quad (1/2)(1/2)^4 = 5/32.$$

Problem 7:

You should get exactly the same answer: 108/256. This time r=3, p=3/4, q=1/4, n=4. That is, exactly 3 successes (normal children) out of 4 children when the probability of a normal child at a single birth is p, 3/4.

Problem 8:

This question is slightly different in that it asks for the probability of *at least* one and not *exactly* one. It requires that you use the addition rule as well as the binomial.

$$P(\text{at least } 1) = P(\text{exactly 1 or exactly 2 or exactly 3}) =$$
$$P(\text{exactly 1}) + P(\text{exactly 2}) + P(\text{exactly 3})$$
since these are mutually exclusive events

$$P(\text{exactly 1}) = \frac{3!}{2!1!} (1/4)^1(3/4)^2 = 27/64$$

$$P(\text{exactly 2}) = \frac{3!}{1!2!} (1/4)^2(3/4)^1 = 9/64$$

$$P(\text{exactly 3}) = \frac{3!}{0!3!} (1/4)^3(3/4)^0 = 1/64$$

Probability of at least one child with Amelogenesis Imperfecta is 37/64, the sum of the three probabilities above. This answer could have also been obtained more directly by noting that

$$P(\text{at least } 1) = 1 - P(\text{less than one}) = 1 - P(\text{zero affected}) =$$

$$1 - \left[\frac{3!}{3!0!} (1/4)^0 (3/4)^3 \right] = 1 - (27/64) = 37/64.$$

POSTTEST 7

After evaluating a panoramic radiograph, Richard's dentist has informed him that he has four impacted third molars and has suggested that he make an appointment with an oral surgeon to have them removed. Richard, however, is an informed consumer and is concerned about unnecessary dental radiography and surgery. He decides to analyze his situation in greater detail before consenting to an irreversible procedure.

Assume that the probability of one of these molars' causing pain or infection in the future is 1/4 and the probability of its remaining unaffected is 3/4. Also assume that the outcome of each molar is independent.

1) What is the probability that *none* of Richard's wisdom teeth will cause a problem in the future?
2) *at least* one will become affected?
3) *exactly* one will become affected?
4) *at most* one will become affected?
5) *all four* will become affected?
6) *exactly two* will become affected?

YOUR ANSWERS TO POSTTEST 7

Name:

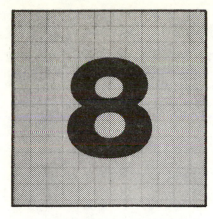

CHAPTER 8

SAMPLING FROM A POPULATION

INTRODUCTION

So far we have seen how data may be described and have been introduced to the idea of probability. We will now go a stage further and learn the methods for relating measurements obtained from a sample to a whole population.

OBJECTIVE

When you finish working through this chapter, you will be able to:
1) Draw a **simple random sample** from a given population, with the aid of a table of **random numbers**;
2) Recognize a given sample as **representative** or **biased,** and give reasons for your choice; and
3) Recognize whether given variables are **discrete** or **continuous**.

A SAMPLE FROM A POPULATION

In your examination of a new patient you measure the systolic blood pressure. This information is of little value unless you can relate it to the distribution of systolic blood pressure for a population that is similar to your patient. Using the population distribution, you should be able to decide whether or not the systolic blood pressure of an individual patient is unusual. However, it is not possible to obtain systolic readings on complete populations and in any case would be excessively expensive. Instead, it is common to select a subset of the population of interest and take measurements on this subset. In statistical language, this subset is called a **sample** and it is important that the sample be representative of the population from which it was drawn. Then statements (or inferences) about the whole population may be made from the measurements taken on the sample.

If a sample is not representative of the population of interest, then it is a **biased** sample. For example, in caries prevalence measures, school children living in a fluoridated community would be a biased sample of all children.

Problem 1:

A health administrator wants to determine what type of dental services are being made available in a neighborhood health center. A clerk is available on Monday, Wednesday and Friday afternoons and for one month he records all the services that are performed at those times.

Is this sample appropriate to determine the types of services being offered?

Your Solution:

SIMPLE RANDOM SAMPLE

When selecting a sample, it is desirable to use some random procedure to determine which items are included in the sample. **A simple random sample is one in which every item in the population has an equal and independent chance of being selected.** For example, a simple random sample of patients in a group practice may be selected by first listing all the patients and numbering them in order. If there were 9500 patients, the numbers would go from 1 to 9500. A table of random numbers, which can be found in many standard statistics textbooks, can then be used to aid in selecting the sample. If a sample of size 500 (i.e., about 5%) is required, then from a random start in the table, sets of 4 consecutive random digits are used to determine the sample. A table of random numbers is usually presented as follows: (read across)

| 83179 | 98001 | 36473 | 87611 |
| 92210 | 06554 | 32879 | 19398 |

i.e., as rows of digits, each row consisting of several groups of five digits. The rows may be split into five groups of four digits as follows:

| 8317/9 | 980/01 | 36/473 | 8/7611 |
| 9221/0 | 065/54 | 32/879 | 1/9398 |

Each set of four digits determines a number in the range 0-9999. The sample of 500 is then determined by reading the sufficient consecutive sets of four digits. Numbers greater than 9500 are ignored. Zero (0000) is ignored and if a 4-digit number is repeated it is also ignored, otherwise a patient might be included in the sample two times. From the random numbers specified, patients numbered 8317, 136, 4738, 7611, 9221, 65, 5432, 8791, 9398 would be included in the sample. Note that the second set of 4 digits (i.e., 9980) is ignored for this sampling procedure, since it represents a number greater than 9500.

If there were more than 10,000 patients in the population of interest, say 15000, then consecutive groups of *five* digits would be used to determine the sample. All numbers up to 15000 can be represented by using 5 digits. In this case all random numbers greater than 15000 would be ignored.

Note: When using a table of random numbers, it is customary to pick a random starting point each time you select a sample. The most elementary way of achieving this random start is to close your eyes and put your finger on a "random" spot in the table.

Problem 2:

Suppose you were interested in the attitudes of dental patients registered with a newly formed HMO. Suppose 848 patients had registered to date and a simple random sample of size 40 was to be selected for interview. Use the following random numbers to determine a simple random sample of patients to be interviewed. Assume the first digit corresponds to a random start.

21648	78245	50328	94107
73186	40021	89707	34583
21054	54581	64310	98980
38219	32728	26434	54329
87373	21019	08372	61486
21324	83649	27384	97101
54872	93612	49581	02001

Your Solution:

OTHER TYPES OF SAMPLES

When selecting a sample based on probabilities, in practice, simple random samples are not used very often. One reason for this is that a simple random sample may allow an unrepresentative sample to be selected, since all possible combinations including unrepresentative ones can occur in a simple random sample. The most common techniques used are equivalent to restricted simple random samples, the restrictions being chosen so that the chances of an unrepresentative sample are minimized. The most common sample of this type is a **stratified random sample** where, for example, steps are taken to assure that selections will be made from each age, sex, race, or social stratum subgroup. There are also non-probability sampling methods, e.g., quota sampling selects the first 10 women or 10 blue collar workers, etc., without regard for the pool that they might represent.

POPULATION DISTRIBUTION

Now, suppose we are sampling from a very large population (e.g., persons living in the United States). If the size of a random sample from a large population is increased and smaller and smaller class intervals are used to construct a histogram for a particular variable, then the histogram will gradually become a smooth curve. The smooth curve represents the **population distribution.** For example, a histogram describing the systolic blood pressure of a sample of young healthy males may look like this:

Figure 8.1

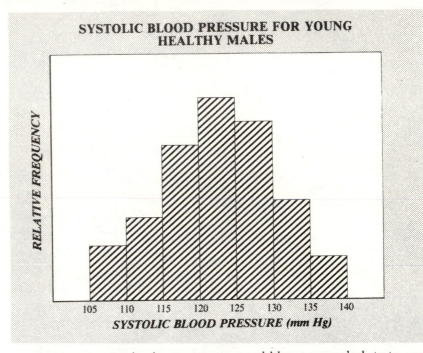

As the sample size increases, we would have enough data to use smaller intervals and the histogram might look as follows.

Figure 8.2

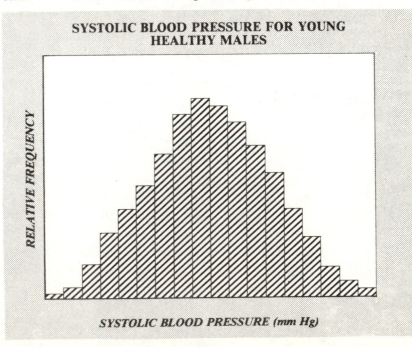

As the sample size gets very large, the histogram would approximate a smooth curve.

Figure 8.3

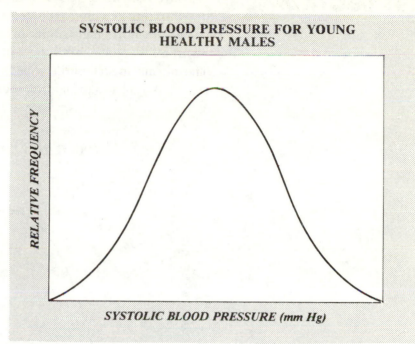

SYSTOLIC BLOOD PRESSURE FOR YOUNG HEALTHY MALES

RELATIVE FREQUENCY

SYSTOLIC BLOOD PRESSURE (mm Hg)

If X is the variable that has been measured (in our example X is systolic blood pressure), then the smooth curve describes the population distribution of the variable X. It is important to realize that population distributions will be smooth curves only for variables which may be *measured* such as blood pressure, height, weight, cholesterol level. In mathematical terminology these are called **continuous variables** since these variables may be measured to any desired degree of accuracy. The only restriction on accuracy is the equipment used and a technician's ability to use the equipment properly.

Continuous variables differ from **discrete variables** in that the latter can only take a restricted set of values. For example the number of assistants employed by a group practice is a discrete variable and the only admissible possibilities are 0, 1, 2, 3,... up to some reasonable maximum, say 10. Discrete variables are described in tables and their population distributions can never be smooth curves. For these variables, their frequency polygons must always remain jagged.

It should be pointed out that continuous variables can be converted to discrete variables if you, the data analyst, wish to do so. In effect, the histogram for a measurement variable does this. Systolic blood pressure is a continuous (measurement) variable but it can be treated as though it were discrete by selecting class intervals and allocating measurements to the appropriate intervals. The converse of this is *not* true; natural discrete variables cannot be converted to continuous variables.

NORMAL DISTRIBUTION

There is one population distribution that occurs very commonly in the life sciences. Several naturally occurring population distributions are approximated very closely by this distribution, namely the **normal distribution.** It is also referred to as the **Gaussian distribution,** named after the famous mathematician J.F.C. Gauss. The normal distribution is bell-shaped and symmetric about its center. A typical normal distribution is shown in Figure 8.4.

Figure 8.4

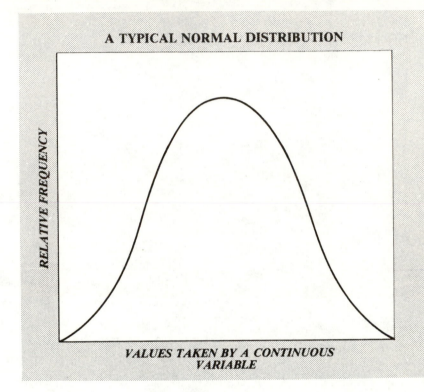

An interesting feature of the normal distribution is that it depends on only two parameters, the population mean μ (mu) and population standard deviation σ (sigma) (see chapter 5). The standard deviation equals the square root of variance. In statistical writings, population parameters are usually represented by Greek letters and should be distinguished from the mean and variance you would calculate from data derived from a sample. In chapter 5, the sample mean was labelled $\bar{x}$, and the sample standard deviation s, using letters of the modern alphabet. These are not population parameters, but quantities derived from a data set which represents only a sample of a population. In chapter 10, you will see how quantities (such as $\bar{x}$ and s) derived from data are used to estimate population parameters (such as μ and σ).

Getting back to the normal distribution, the mean μ determines where the peak of the curve is located and the standard deviation σ determines how spread out or concentrated the distribution is. Figure 8.5 shows 3 normal distributions with the same mean, but different standard deviations.

Figure 8.5

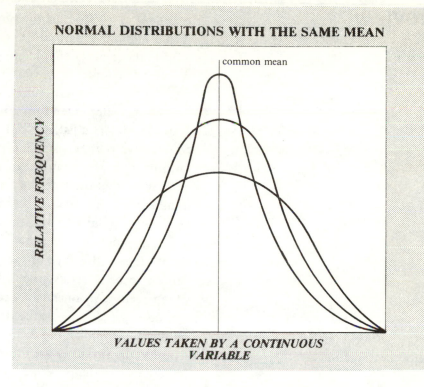

The more spread out the curve, the larger the standard deviation, that is, the greater the variability in the data set.

Figure 8.6 shows three normal distributions with the same standard deviation (σ), but different means μ_1. μ_2, μ_3.

Figure 8.6

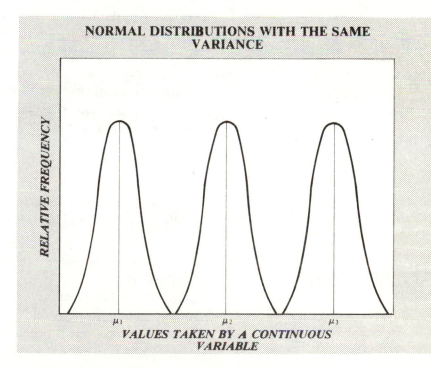

In the next chapter you will see how to calculate probabilities under the normal distribution using statistical tables.

REVIEW

1) A **sample** is a subset of the population being investigated.

2) A **representative sample** is a subset of the population which reflects the general characteristics of that population.

3) A **biased sample** is a subset of the population that is not representative of the population as a whole.

4) To obtain a **simple random sample** you first decide on the size of your sample. You list and give each member of the population a consecutive number, starting from 1. Then, by using a table of random numbers, you select consecutive random numbers to determine the ones to be included in the sample, ignoring numbers that are repeated and also ignoring all numbers larger than the population size, together with zero.

   Remember that, in practice, simple random samples are not used often, as this type of sample will allow an unrepresentative sample to be selected, since all possible combinations including unrepresentative ones can occur. The most common practical technique used is a stratified random sample, the strata being chosen to minimize the chances of unrepresentativeness.

5) **Continuous variables** are those variables which can be measured to any desired degree of accuracy, the only restrictions being the accuracy of the equipment used and the ability of the technician using the measuring instruments. Examples of these variables are blood pressure, height, weight, and cholesterol level. Population distributions of these variables may be described by smooth curves.

6) **Discrete variables** can take only a restricted set of values, for example the number of teeth present or missing. A discrete variable is limited in number of categories by some reasonable maximum, for example 0, 1, 2, . . . up to 32 teeth. Population distributions of discrete variables are not smooth curves; the frequency polygons depicting these variables are always jagged.

7) The **normal distribution** is a **population distribution** which appears very commonly in life sciences. It is bell shaped, symmetrical about its center and depends on only two parameters:
   a) the population **mean,** (mu), symbolized by μ.
   b) the population **standard deviation,** (sigma), symbolized by σ.

SOLUTIONS

Problem 1:

No. It is likely that different types of patients are treated at different times of the day. More pedodontic services may be rendered in the afternoons if the clinic is primarily visited by children during those hours. Adults who cannot leave their places of employment during the day are more likely to utilize evening hours and Saturdays. Thus, more prosthetic and endodontic services may be rendered during evening and weekend hours.

The sample should include representation from all the hours that the practice is open.

Problem 2:

The 848 patients must be listed in a numerical order so that each patient has a different number in the range 1-848. This ordering can be done in any way. *Three* random digits will determine a number in the range 0-999 and this is convenient since we have a population of 848 (848 has 3 digits). The random numbers should be split into sets of 3 digits as follows:

216/48	7/824/5	50/328/	941/07
7/318/6	40/021/	897/07	3/458/3
21/054/	545/81	6/431/0	98/980/
382/19	3/272/8	26/434/	543/29
8/737/3	21/019/	083/72	6/148/6
21/324/	836/49	2/738/4	97/101
548/72	9/361/2	49/581/	020/01

The consecutive sets of 3 digits may be used to determine the 40 patients in the sample. These will be patients numbered 216, 487, 824, 550, 328, 77, 318, 640, 21, 73, 458, 321, 54, 545, 816, 431, 98, 382, 193, 272, 826, 434, 543, 298, 737, 19, 83, 726, 148, 621, 324, 836, 492, 738, 497, 101, 548, 729, 361, 249. Note that 321 appears twice and was omitted on the second occasion; and 941, 897, and 980 were ignored because they were greater than 848.

POSTTEST 8

A dental hygienist practicing in a Veterans Administration Hospital is interested in developing a program of preventive care and early non-surgical treatment for all the potential periodontal patients in the medical center. She feels the need for some preliminary information about all patients who are at risk of periodontitis. She asks a friend who teaches biostatistics at a local university to help her obtain this preliminary information. The professor assesses the situation and then sends a graduate student to carry out the procedures. The student selected a simple random sample of 20 patients from a list of 300 patients, aged 55-80, who were being treated at the V.A. Hospital. This list had been constructed a few months previously, for a study of the relationship between stress and periodontal disease.

Assume you are the graduate student conducting this research. On the next two pages is the list of 300 names. On the page following the last sheet of names is a reproduction of a table of random numbers with a portion of the numbers outlined.

1) Take a simple random sample of 20 patients from the 300 patient population using the table of random numbers. Assume the first digit of the portion outlined corresponds to a random start in the

table. List the numbers of the 20 patients chosen for inclusion in the sample.

2) Recall that the hygienist was interested in all potential periodontal patients. Is the sample selected representative of all potential periodontal patients?

3) When a study deals with variables such as the *number of auxiliary personnel in Massachusetts HMOs*, what type of variable is being considered?

4) When studying *blood pressure, height*, and *weight*, what type of variable is under consideration? Are there any *restrictions* on the accuracy of measurements?

LIST OF 300 PATIENTS AGED 55-80 IN A VETERANS ADMINISTRATION HOSPITAL

1. James Adams	46. Wilbert Camp	91. Conrad Gailey
2. Elwin Adderton	47. Haskell Campbell	92. Harold Gaines
3. William Agee	48. Floyd Campbell	93. Simon Gaines
4. Larry Aiken	49. George Campbell	94. Leonard Gallimore
5. Frank Albertson	50. Bobby Canada	95. Stokes Gallimore
6. Carl Albritton	51. Elmer Canada	96. Linnel Haas
7. Floyd Aldridge	52. Milton Cannon	97. Bob Hackler
8. James Alford	53. Jimmy Canoy	98. Walt Hackler
9. Bob Allen	54. William Dabbs	99. Neil Hadley
10. Kevin Allen	55. Francis Dailey	100. Mickey Hager
11. Junior Allgood	56. Robert Dailey	101. Glen Hagie
12. Bob Alston	57. Veirgis Damron	102. Val Hailey
13. William Alston	58. Richard Daniel	103. Daniel Hair
14. Willie Alston	59. Mel Daniels	104. Ben Hair
15. Jose Alvarez	60. Joe Daughtridge	105. Francis Hairston
16. Bill Amos	61. Sam Eaddy	106. Oscar Haithcock
17. Harold Amos	62. Harry Earle	107. Royce Haithcock
18. Chester Anderson	63. Virgil Early	108. Roy Iddings
19. Eugene Babb	64. Merle Earp	109. Gary Iddings
20. Norton Bacon	65. Larry East	110. Charles Idol
21. Chester Baffa	66. Egbert Easter	111. Edd Idol
22. Joseph Bailes	67. Clearence Eaton	112. Oscar Ijames
23. Ross Bailey	68. Kyle Eccles	113. Dennis Ijames
24. Thomas Bain	69. Edward Echerd	114. Marvin Ikerd
25. Donald Bain	70. Lewis Eckert	115. Lauren Ikerd
26. Phil Baisey	71. John Edge	116. Eugene Ikner
27. Fred Baker	72. Baxter Fain	117. Davis Ilderton
28. Timothy Baker	73. Clifford Fain	118. Leroy Ingle
29. Leroy Baker	74. Niles Faircloth	119. Pat Ingle ·
30. Len Baker	75. Willie Faircloth	120. Horace Jackson
31. Carl Baldwin	76. Lou Fallenstein	121. Albert Jackson
32. Dale Baldwin	77. Azlee Falls	122. Dan Jackson
33. Billy Balkcum	78. Andy Farlow	123. David Jackson
34. Eller Ball	79. Arnold Farlow	124. Billy Jacobs
35. Henry Bame	80. Howard Farlow	125. Cal Jacobs
36. Lance Bame	81. Clarence Farmer	126. Robert Jacobs
37. Darrell Cable	82. Daniel Feemster	127. Earton James
38. Barney Cagle	83. Brady Felts	128. Baxter James
39. Bill Cain	84. Lister Gabriel	129. William James
40. Cale Cain	85. David Gadd	130. Claude Jarrell
41. James Calhoun	86. Eddy Gaddy	131. Jim Jarrell
42. Walter Calloway	87. John Gaddy	132. Julian Kabat
43. Ted Calomiris	88. Ross Gaddy	133. Richard Kalte
44. Carmel Cambareri	89. Richmond Gage	134. Gary Kaney
45. Bob Cameron	90. Riley Gahagan	135. Himler Kanter

136. Matty Kasias	191. Mack O'Kelly	246. Joseph Sanborn
137. Michael Katz	192. Mel Pace	247. James Sanborn
138. Mitchell Keahey	193. Joseph Packer	248. Jack Sanford
139. Amos Kearns	194. Edgar Padgett	249. Robert Sandman
140. Bond Kearns	195. Fate Fadgett	250. Greg Saunders
141. Heywood Keaton	196. Ernest Page	251. Frazier Saunders
142. Edwin Keenan	197. Vance Page	252. Douglas Sawyer
143. Clarence Keever	198. Bill Palmer	253. Kenneth Sawyer
144. James Lacey	199. Gene Pardue	254. Chuck Scarboro
145. Heath Lacey	200. Donald Parham	255. Willie Scarboro
146. Donald Lackey	201. Jay Paris	256. Alden Scarce
147. Lester Lackey	201. Frank Paris	257. Leonard Scarce
148. David Lacy	203. Andrew Parker	258. Allard Schnell
149. Zeke Lacy	204. Frank Queen	259. Gerald Schoen
150. Albert Larkins	205. Jack Queen	260. Carroll Stirewalt
151. Paul Larkins	206. Lonnie Quesenberry	261. Joe Stockton
152. Charles Lambert	207. Alan Quesenberry	262. Clement Stokes
153. Billy Lambeth	208. Cleveland Quick	263. James Stokes
154. Robert Lamb	209. Cal Quick	264. Tom Stone
155. Zack Lamb	210. Elijah Quicker	265. Robert Stone
156. John Lampe	211. Max Quicker	266. Igor Stout
157. Jared Land	212. Stancil Quigley	267. James Stout
158. David Maas	213. Martin Quigley	268. Milt Stratton
159. Heck Maas	214. Hall Quinn	269. Rolland Stratton
160. Dewey Mabe	215. Burton Quinn	270. Jerry Streeter
161. Enoch Mabe	216. Morton Rabhan	271. Charles Stribling
162. Garry Mabry	217. Ich Rabon	272. Ed Strickland
163. Vern Mabry	218. Ronnie Rabon	273. Clarence Strickland
164. Louis MacAluso	219. Rob Raby	274. Bertie Stroud
165. Clay Mack	220. James Raby	275. James Tabor
166. Alan MacKeraghan	221. Karl Ragan	276. Silas Tackett
167. Ken MacKeraghan	222. Herbert Ragland	277. Miles Talbert
168. Tyree Nabors	223. Lon Ragsdale	278. Francis Talton
169. Bert Nalley	224. Thomas Rahsdale	279. Harry Tanner
170. John Nalley	225. Phil Rains	280. Mittie Tate
171. Bart Nance	226. Floyd Rains	281. Roger Tate
172. Jack Nance	227. Macy Rakocy	282. Arnie Taylor
173. Robert Nance	228. Grady Saferight	283. Buddy Taylor
174. Roger Nance	229. Leon Safrit	284. Gary Taylor
175. George Nash	230. Bennie Saintsing	285. Carlyle Teague
176. Paul Nash	231. Bernie Sale	286. Royce Teague
177. Hal Newman	232. Nelson Sale	287. Clyde Teal
178. Jim Newman	233. Stokes Salley	288. Ron Teal
179. Nick Newsome	234. Terry Salley	289. James Tedder
180. Charles Oakley	235. Bill Salters	290. Desmond Teeter
181. Peter Oakley	236. Allie Salway	291. Joe Temple
182. Patrick O'Brien	237. Mose Samet	292. Elton Terrell
183. Niles Ockershauser	238. Nestor Samet	293. Tom Terrell
184. Jerry Odell	239. Edward Sampson	294. Philip Terry
185. Mark Odell	240. Izzy Sampson	295. Randall Terry
186. James Odum	241. Bobby Sampson	296. Rhodes Tharp
187. Gilbert Odum	242. Edwin Sams	297. Banks Thayer
188. Herbert Oglesby	243. Jacob Sams	298. Ed Thomas
189. Adam O'Ham	244. Andy Samuel	299. Frank Thomas
190. George O'Ham	245. Robert Samuel	300. Paul Thomas

TABLE OF 3000 RANDOM DIGITS
****

```
59559  72852  06129  94308  05749  19153  82460  00478  75805  32009  23875  68677
82411  90292  30706  97605  18608  54015  51890  17301  99782  19015  57317  68013
13843  93995  51883  58522  61155  71399  59635  85023  51650  76718  21919  73513
10435  78326  64618  93437  07475  30624  38191  55187  35325  94395  73433  94676
53134  66704  32257  59501  47700  00009  06281  98418  76171  96940  09059  69417
72003  34132  73190  69210  97567  74020  66713  12659  93589  94662  43405  10066
28514  51642  08530  95539  05602  63012  18957  88944  94453  93122  64781  06514
12917  97462  25726  94744  35448  13042  50943  79709  67889  29609  62313  79279
83373  39245  92243  97913  17124  85041  85635  45813  53811  37392  24970  79927
07267  86897  51499  43273  18892  82216  80236  57612  14001  62325  38735  84612
76588  26923  31054  60218  17345  39602  59162  57832  84523  43042  11296  30632
49240  63281  04614  33392  07001  84306  16429  53471  25818  63352  46924  04871
35752  04189  94171  14157  74892  95415  33440  30640  51485  68458  10328  33676
64619  77118  41617  30554  18276  44883  99415  16997  53821  94097  75026  81127
88690  61236  33374  60728  14229  29563  34529  88056  68232  68392  76796  55893
79461  84305  43579  72883  38477  67290  94245  99781  10942  80435  00921  14067
80902  36897  95640  35470  62245  03058  08547  50958  83273  19123  09752  08407
01157  21104  97521  58900  05404  06173  80832  51058  85639  39027  46466  51809
37958  64462  56075  08893  37611  99308  04329  93183  30336  21644  58715  38198
23305  26085  92374  32990  26363  91711  69860  05770  29751  97144  07013  86938
59247  16366  96189  97470  30214  44644  98059  22574  91620  60000  23344  37444
36500  60822  90378  97279  23465  08334  02857  55667  47936  56996  89202  83199
70075  54440  64481  84409  41831  60664  47231  82181  43874  30630  26199  45896
86342  24223  44496  59162  48388  74147  98995  81431  34897  34988  36418  02624
84311  88398  64297  44436  58368  20076  99158  96858  50086  65045  38481  07525
54881  63813  61062  90259  29431  43074  28667  69796  93533  22809  99394  69098
14518  41841  98054  66992  22445  17229  43071  14225  88268  00541  71165  14783
50638  67367  02269  41450  41821  68571  23399  93457  89750  57769  21497  89342
69344  86839  20010  07328  29007  80903  54847  30916  17892  82137  53555  20075
47913  28647  19802  76446  97037  70494  69812  09447  32454  42213  09634  72966
26328  57898  18788  24756  85277  52756  63983  56075  33968  14871  02049  60706
50294  16119  83076  90665  84829  49972  46220  16659  46931  92976  65504  06336
83268  99346  59662  48680  42779  03996  94530  98456  01265  74255  91891  12575
07013  87702  50796  70856  97815  32459  12438  76268  47025  97690  79257  36095
46765  50390  54010  78801  07072  98988  33444  99065  94077  10472  23690  92832
08395  47064  95976  87412  70468  75482  08605  29299  35481  73600  64300  33511
60885  24370  73993  25812  84663  70534  56393  53047  35756  69593  79344  90015
27015  06788  34710  77319  00486  64682  87293  41380  21570  14220  87665  74506
00315  92095  71436  53910  71825  35262  29177  02301  62587  61783  55570  55539
53950  65678  20747  31728  09918  25385  77090  01288  94658  74075  88671  49665
99690  59155  81227  47763  47492  04772  94845  40646  56216  21067  42450  19508
66717  11954  01415  45326  51054  42341  34358  85431  83353  87605  36601  06658
26188  30485  81426  23423  23594  09460  41692  05812  82406  15391  35229  17837
90362  41289  37152  07100  23518  50267  32448  62141  01385  36778  27664  59578
82823  69136  09321  04700  63892  27441  67295  65525  52824  23557  96270  69621
42577  06630  63342  07561  50529  70119  79646  51437  92659  13088  04551  00541
23822  36622  50194  18562  02049  10746  05935  51914  76822  08605  11330  73731
32678  80671  56245  21450  03647  04769  21619  45623  61887  83380  85757  41796
23175  01870  06887  58787  91034  07951  98761  15623  11588  16364  82436  89947
10889  22960  89466  62824  01679  49788  03503  79381  92170  16860  46220  73179
```

YOUR ANSWERS
TO POSTTEST 8

Name:

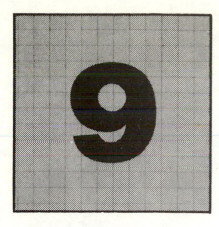

CHAPTER 9

THE NORMAL DISTRIBUTION

INTRODUCTION

In the last chapter you were introduced by name to the **normal distribution,** and were shown its shape as follows:

Figure 9.1

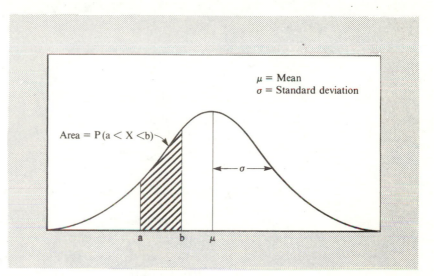

While the normal distribution is only one of many kinds of continuous probability distributions, it is a very widely applicable one, perhaps the most widely applicable of any in the life sciences. Consequently, it is very important that you understand this distribution and are able to calculate the probabilities associated with it.

OBJECTIVE

The overall objective of this chapter is to calculate the probability that an event or phenomenon will fall within a specified range of values. The values that occur are governed by a normal distribution with mean (μ) and standard deviation (σ). These probabilities are calculated by using a standard normal distribution. In particular, you will be able to:

1) Calculate probabilities using the standard normal distribution,

2) Translate a given question about a normal distribution into a

corresponding question about the standard normal distribution.
3) Calculate the probabilities for any normal distribution.

THE STANDARD NORMAL DISTRIBUTION

The **standard normal distribution** is the normal distribution in which **the mean is zero and the standard deviation is one:** $\mu=0$, $\sigma=1$. It has become customary to use the letter capital Z to designate the variable associated with this distribution. Z denotes the variable name, and small letter z denotes the value taken by Z. Z may take any positive or negative value, and the probability with which it takes particular values is governed by the shape of the curve of the standard normal distribution.

Figure 9.2

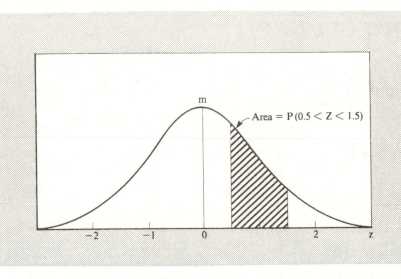

Tables have been prepared to enable us to read the areas under the standard normal curve. Various tables are constructed in various different formats. One that is used often is attached at the end of this chapter. It is labeled *The Standard Normal Distribution,* and it gives the area to the left of a point on the z axis, for a large number of values of z.

Figure 9.3

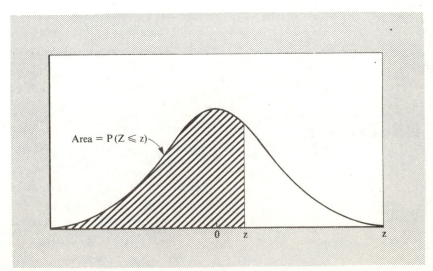

For example, the probability that Z be equal to or less than 0.5, that is the area under the standard normal curve to the left of $z = 0.5$, can be found by entering the table with $z = 0.5$ and reading .6915:

Figure 9.4

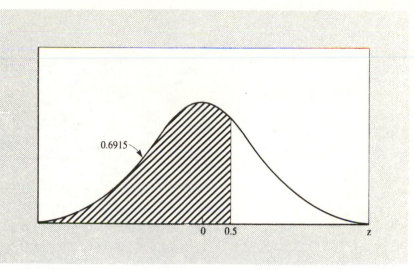

Problem 1:

Try it yourself. What is the probability that Z has a value not exceeding -1.2?

Your Solution:

Please note that to look up a negative value of z in the table at the end of this chapter, you look up the z value as though it were positive and then you subtract from unity the probability value in the table.

Remember that a probability gives both the likelihood that a single random drawing from a population has the specified property, and also the proportion (or fraction) of the entire population which *has* that property. For example, in a standard normal population, 40% of the members of the population have z-measurements equal to or less than -0.253:

Figure 9.5

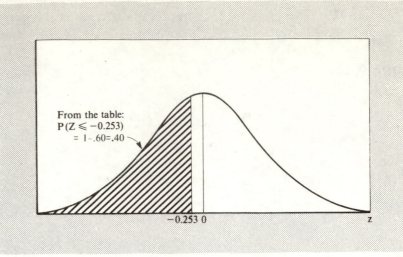

From the table:
$P(Z \leqslant -0.253)$
$= 1 - .60 = .40$

Notice that having 40% of the standard normal population with z-values equal to or less than -0.253 means also that *60%* of that population has z-values *larger than* -0.253.

Problem 2:

For your own example, find the fraction of a standard normal population which has measurements in excess of 2.0.

Your Solution:

From this you can begin to see the way we maneuver to produce the probability for any kind of interval of z-values. We use the table to give us total area to the left of any z-value we like, and subtract areas as necessary to give us the area we want. For example, let us find the probability that Z will lie between -0.4 and +1.3. The table and the following diagram give us the answer.

Figure 9.6

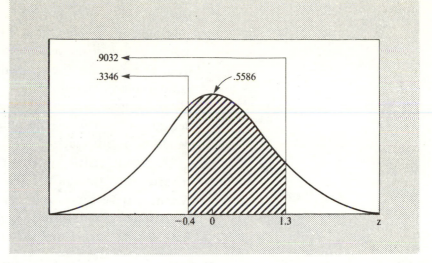

The total area to the left of +1.3 is .9032, and the total area to the left of -0.4 is .3446. Therefore, the area *between* the two values must be .9032 - .3446 = .5586.

Problem 3:

You can now produce the value for the probability shown by area in Figure 9.2: P(0.5 < Z < 1.5).

Your Solution:

Now that you can produce probabilities at will in the standard normal distribution, you need only learn a small translation formula which transforms any normal distribution into a *standard* normally distributed Z. Perfectly proper mathematical theory has produced the fact that, if X has the normal distribution with mean μ and standard deviation σ, then the fraction $(X-\mu)/\sigma$ has the standard normal distribution; in other words, we can use the translation formula:

$$\frac{(X-\mu)}{\sigma} = Z$$

A young patient comes into an orthodontist's office with his mother. Anthony's mother is concerned because his teeth are crowded and wants to know if he will need braces. Before making a diagnosis, the orthodontist wants to take impressions of Anthony's teeth and examine the resulting models as well as analyze several radiographic views of Anthony's dentition and skull. It is necessary to carefully measure the widths of Anthony's permanent and deciduous teeth before deciding if a program of serial extraction would be appropriate.

A recent article in Dr. Y. R. Bender's orthodontic journal reported that the normal distribution of maxillary central incisor widths can be represented by a mean of 8.5mm and a standard deviation of .5mm. If we designate X = central incisor width, then we have $\mu = 8.5$, $\sigma = .5$ and the conversion formula is:

$$\frac{X - 8.5}{.5} = Z$$

Figure 9.7

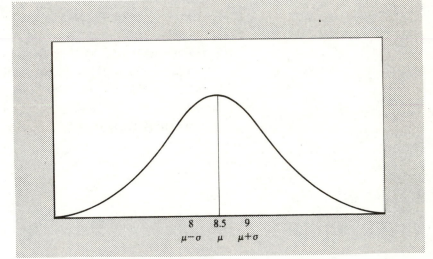

If a central incisor measured 9.5mm, would you say that this is a particularly large tooth? What fraction of maxillary central incisors have widths *as large as* 9.5mm? That is, what is $P(X \geqslant 9.5)$?

If this were a question about Z, we could at once go to the table and in a moment or so come up with the answer we want. Now we have to translate, knowing that the conversion formula tells us that we get a Z whenever we subtract μ from X and divide by σ. In our question about tooth size, both the X and 9.5 are X values, so we shall translate them both. Also remember that in this case $\mu = 8.5$ and $\sigma = .5$.

So we have the following:

$$P(X \geqslant 9.5)$$

$$= P\left[\frac{(X-8.5)}{.5} \geqslant \frac{(9.5-8.5)}{.5}\right]$$

$$= P\left[Z \geqslant \frac{(9.5 - 8.5)}{.5}\right]$$

$$= P\left[Z \geqslant \frac{1.0}{.5} \right]$$
$$= P\,(Z \geqslant 2.0)$$

From here we go to the table and get the entry for giving us the answer:

$$P(Z \geqslant 2.0) = 1 - .9773 = .0227$$

That is 2.27% of central incisors in this population are 9.5mm wide or wider. If this was an elderly patient requiring a denture, and the dental supply companies felt that this tooth size was unusually large, you might have difficulty obtaining the appropriate size denture tooth for this patient.

Problem 4:

You received a grade of 86 on a BIOSTATS post test. The scores for your class can be considered as having a normal distribution, with a mean grade of 82 and a standard deviation of 8. Where do you stand in the class regarding your performance on this test?

Your Solution:

Problem 5:

What is the probability that a student drawn at random from the class would have received a grade less than 70?

Your Solution:

It is just a bit more work to deal with intervals closed in on both sides. What is the probability that a student from the class chosen at random would have received a grade between 66 and 94?

$$P (66 < X < 94)$$

$$= P \left[\frac{(66\text{-}82)}{8} < \frac{(X\text{-}82)}{8} < \frac{(94\text{-}82)}{8} \right]$$

$$= P \left[\frac{\text{-}16}{8} < Z < \frac{12}{8} \right]$$

$$= P (\text{-}2.0 < Z < 1.5)$$

$$= .9332 - .0227 = .9105$$

Figure 9.8

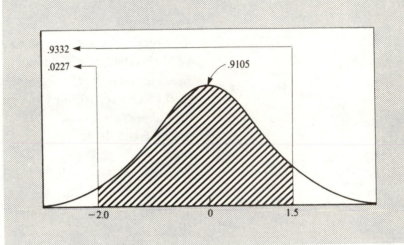

Problem 6:

In a certain dental school, the amount of weight that the students gain between their first day of school and graduation is normally distributed with a mean of five pounds and a standard deviation of 2 pounds.

What is the probability that a student chosen at random will gain between 6 and 11 pounds?

What proportion of dental students *lose* weight during their years in dental school?

Your Solution:

STANDARD DEVIATIONS

Figure 9.9

One final item: It is useful to remember the proportion of measurements which fall within one, two, or three standard deviations of the mean for a normal distribution with mean μ and standard deviation σ.

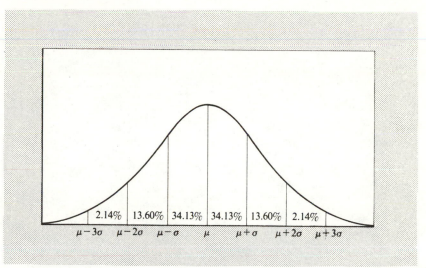

For a normal distribution the following statements hold:

1) **68.26%** (= 34.13% + 34.13%) of the population lies **within one** standard deviation of the mean.
2) **95.46%** (= 34.13% + 34.13% + 13.60% + 13.60%) of the population lies **within two** standard deviations of the mean.
3) **99.74%** (= 34.13% + 34.13% + 13.60% + 13.60% + 2.14% + 2.14%) of the population lies **within three** standard deviations of the mean.

Usually, statement 2 is approximated to be as follows:

95% of a normal population lie within two standard deviations of the mean.

Statements 1, 2 and 3 can be seen easily by referring to the table on the standard normal distribution.

We consider a normal distribution with mean μ and standard deviation σ. The values that can be taken by individuals in the population are denoted by X.

Statement 1:
We require that X lies in the range μ-σ, μ+σ.

$$P\left[(\mu\text{-}\sigma) < X < (\mu\text{+}\sigma) \right]$$
$$= P\left[\frac{(\mu\text{-}\sigma) - \mu}{\sigma} < Z < \frac{(\mu\text{+}\sigma) - \mu}{\sigma} \right]$$
$$= P\left[\frac{-\sigma}{\sigma} < Z < \frac{\sigma}{\sigma} \right]$$
$$= P(-1 < Z < 1)$$
$$= 0.8413 - 0.1587 = 0.6826$$

i.e., 68.26% of the population lies within one standard deviation of the mean.

Problem 7:
Show that statements 2 and 3 are correct.

Your Solution:

SOLUTIONS

Figure 9.10

Problem 1:
Translate "not exceeding" as "equal to or less than" and enter the table where z = 1.2, using $P(Z \leqslant -1.2) = 1 - P(Z \leqslant 1.2) = 1 - .8849 = .1151$:

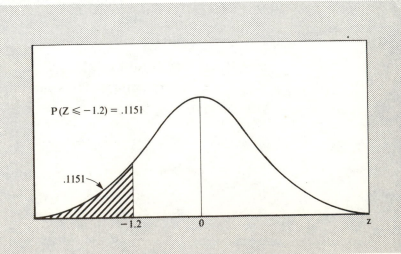

Problem 2:

If all went well, you entered the table with x=2.0, read $P(Z \leq 2.0) = .9773$, and from that reasoned that $P(Z > 2.0) = 1 - .9773 = .0227$, giving 2.27% as the fraction of the population having z-measurements larger than 2.0.

Figure 9.11

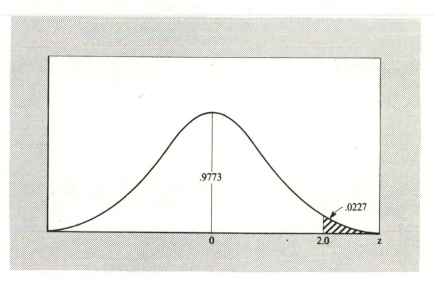

Problem 3:

Figure 9.12

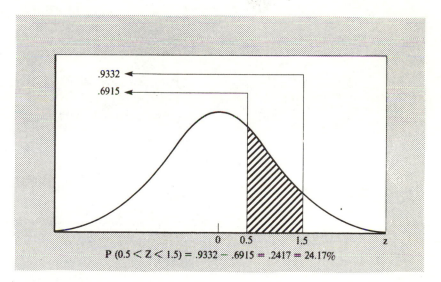

$P(0.5 < Z < 1.5) = .9332 - .6915 = .2417 = 24.17\%$

Problem 4:

$$Z = (86-82/8) = 4/8 = .5$$

Your performance is 1/2 standard deviation above the mean performance. Looking at the table, you can determine that your grade was higher than 69.15% of the class.

Problem 5:

P (X < 70)

$$= P \left[\frac{(X-82)}{8} < \frac{(70-82)}{8} \right]$$

= P (Z < -12/8)

= P (Z < -1.5)

= .0668 or 6.68%

Figure 9.13

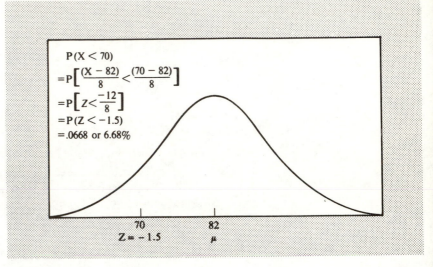

Problem 6:

X = weight gain (lbs.) during dental school

X is normally distributed, μ = 5, σ = 2

$$= P \left[\frac{(6-5)}{2} < \frac{(X-5)}{2} < \frac{(11-5)}{2} \right]$$

= P (1/2 < Z < 6/2)

= P (.5 < Z < 3)

= .9987 - .6915 = .3072

30.72% of the students will gain between 6 and 11 lbs.

Figure 9.14

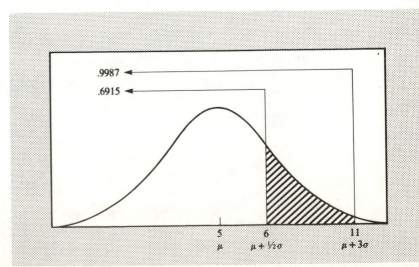

If a student loses weight, then the weight gain is negative, that is $x < 0$. Then we must find $P(X < 0)$.

$$P(X < 0)$$

$$= P\left[\frac{(X-5)}{2} < \frac{(0-5)}{2}\right]$$

$$= P(Z < -5/2)$$

$$= P(Z < -2.5) = .0062$$

.62% of the students lose weight.

Problem 7:
Statement 2:

We require X lies in the range $\mu - 2\sigma$, $\mu + 2\sigma$

$$P\left[\frac{(\mu-2\sigma)-\mu}{\sigma} < Z < \frac{(\mu+2\sigma)-\mu}{\sigma}\right]$$

$$= P(-2\sigma/\sigma < Z < 2\sigma/\sigma)$$

$$= P(-2 < Z < 2)$$

$$= 0.9773 - 0.0227 = 0.9546$$

i.e., 95.46% of the population lies within two standard deviations of the mean.

Statement 3:

We require X lies in the range $\mu - 3\sigma$, $\mu + 3\sigma$.

$$= P\left[\frac{(\mu-3\sigma)-\mu}{\sigma} < Z < \frac{(\mu+3\sigma)-\mu}{\sigma}\right]$$

$$= P(-3\sigma/\sigma < Z < 3\sigma/\sigma)$$

$$= P(-3 < Z < 3)$$

$$= 0.9987 - 0.0013 = 0.9974$$

i.e., 99.74% of the population lies within 3 standard deviations of the mean.

POSTTEST 9

A survey of dentists in a certain state showed that the number of hours per week in patient contact was normally distributed with a mean of 33.5 hours and a standard deviation of 2.5 hours.

1) What proportion of this dentist population spend in the range of 30-35 hours/week actually seeing patients?

2) What proportion of this dentist population spend at least 40 hours/week in patient contact?

THE STANDARD NORMAL DISTRIBUTION

z	P(Z<z)	z	P(Z<z)	z	P(Z<z)	z	P(Z<z)
0.0000	0.5000	0.8416	0.8000	1.6000	0.9452	2.4000	0.9918
0.1000	0.5398	0.9000	0.8159	1.6450	0.9500	2.5000	0.9938
0.1257	0.5500	1.0000	0.8413	1.7000	0.9554	2.5760	0.9950
0.2000	0.5793	1.0364	0.8500	1.7510	0.9600	2.6000	0.9953
0.2533	0.6000	1.1000	0.8643	1.8000	0.9641	2.7000	0.9965
0.3000	0.6179	1.2000	0.8849	1.8810	0.9700	2.8000	0.9974
0.3853	0.6500	1.2816	0.9000	1.9000	0.9713	2.9000	0.9981
0.4000	0.6554	1.3000	0.9032	1.9600	0.9750	3.0000	0.9987
0.5000	0.6915	1.3410	0.9100	2.0000	0.9773	3.0900	0.9990
0.5244	0.7000	1.4000	0.9192	2.0540	0.9800	3.2000	0.9993
0.6000	0.7257	1.4050	0.9200	2.1000	0.9821	3.2910	0.9995
0.6745	0.7500	1.4760	0.9300	2.2000	0.9861	3.4000	0.9997
0.7000	0.7580	1.5000	0.9332	2.3000	0.9893	3.6000	0.9998
0.8000	0.7881	1.5550	0.9400	2.3260	0.9900	3.7190	0.9999

For negative quantities $-z$, use $P(Z \leq -z) = 1 - P(Z < z)$

YOUR ANSWERS TO POSTTEST 9

Name:

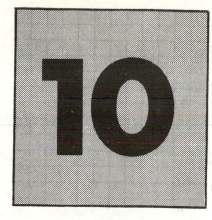

CHAPTER 10

ESTIMATION

INTRODUCTION

If we wanted to know what the overall oral hygiene status was of a certain population residing on a small, remote island in the Pacific, we could theoretically examine the entire population, determine their score on the simplified oral hygiene index, OHI-S, and calculate the mean score or other appropriate measure of central tendency that was discussed in chapter 5. However, this would be highly impractical if we were studying a large population such as the one in the United States. Instead, we try to select and examine a sample of the population that is representative of the entire population. If we selected more than one sample, each one is likely to be a little bit different, each with its own mean and standard deviation. Fortunately, we can circumvent this problem and still make inferences about the entire population from our one sample because of a mathematical result called the **central limit theorem.**

OBJECTIVES

1) You will be able to state the central limit theorem.
2) You will be able to calculate the sample mean and standard error of the sample mean for any sample of observations taken from a population.
3) You will be able to calculate and interpret confidence intervals.

CENTRAL LIMIT THEOREM

Suppose from a population we could select all possible random samples of size n and compute the mean, $\bar{x}$, for each sample, Now, using the means computed for each of these samples, the $\bar{x}$'s, we could calculate an overall mean utilizing these sample means. The mean for *all* the sample means is equivalent to the mean for the entire population:

$$\bar{x}_{\bar{x}} = \mu$$

The standard deviation of all the $\bar{x}$'s is $\sigma/\sqrt{n}$, where "n" refers to the size or number of observations in each sample. This is called the **Standard Error** of the sample mean:

$$SE(\bar{x}) = \sigma_{\bar{x}} = \sigma/\sqrt{n}$$

The standard error of the sample mean depends on the amount of variability in the population and the size of the sample. However, the underlying population does not need to have a normal distribution for the distribution of the sample means to be expressed in the terms which up to now we have been using to describe a *normal* population. The individual observations, the x's, may have any type of frequency distribution. The distribution of *means* of samples from the population will look like a normal distribution. As the sample size, n, increases, it looks more and more like the normal distribution.

The central limit theorem states that the distribution of means, x̄'s, of samples of size n taken from a distribution of almost any shape with mean μ, and standard deviation, σ, approaches a normal distribution with mean μ, and standard deviation $\sigma / \sqrt{n}$.

Figure 10.1

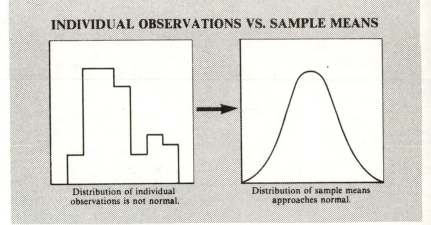

INDIVIDUAL OBSERVATIONS VS. SAMPLE MEANS

Distribution of individual observations is not normal.

Distribution of sample means approaches normal.

As investigators, we do not want to take many samples from a population. We would like to be able to take only one sample. How does the central limit theorem help us?

In previous chapters, you have learned how to calculate the sample variance, s^2, and mean, x̄, from a single random sample containing n observations. The true variance, σ^2/n, of the approximately normal distribution of sample means may be estimated by s^2/n. This sample variance of the distribution of sample means, which one can calculate from the data collected in only one sample, is designated: $s_{\bar{x}}^2$. Thus, the approximated variance of sample means = $s_{\bar{x}}^2 = s^2/n$. Similarly, the approximated standard error of the mean based on a sample instead of a whole population is:

$$SE = s_{\bar{x}} = \sqrt{(s^2/n)} = s/\sqrt{n}$$

Using the results stated above, we are in a position to say something about the distribution of means of other samples of this size without actually taking further samples.

Problem 1:

If 25 random samples from the Boston, Massachusetts population were selected, each containing 400 individuals, and the oral hygiene scores were recorded for these individuals, what would be the distribution of the mean OHI-S scores for these 25 samples?

Your Solution:

Problem 2:
If the variance of one of the samples is .36, what is the estimated standard error for the mean based on this sample?

Your Solution:

To review, the distribution of means of random samples of size n taken from almost any distribution having unknown mean, μ, and standard deviation, σ, is approximately normal with mean equal to the unknown population μ and a standard deviation, $\sigma/\sqrt{n}$, which may be approximated by $s_{\overline{x}} = s/\sqrt{n}$.

From your study of normal distributions in chapter 9, you learned that 95% of the area in a normal distribution falls within approximately two standard deviations on either side of the mean. Similarly, 95% of the distribution of sample means will lie within 2 $\sigma/\sqrt{n}$ units on either side of μ, or within the interval $\mu \pm 2 \sigma/\sqrt{n}$. Unfortunately, in most instances the true population variance σ^2 is unknown. Fortunately, for fairly large sample sizes ($n \geqslant 30$) we may use our approximate variance s^2 in place of the unknown variance σ^2 and say that 95% of the time the true mean, μ, will be spanned by the interval:

$$\overline{x} \pm 2s_{\overline{x}} = \overline{x} \pm 2s/\sqrt{n}.$$

This leads us to confidence intervals.

CONFIDENCE INTERVALS

Unless our sample includes the entire population, we will never know the value of μ, but only have an estimate of the value of μ. We would like to pin down the value of μ within some range and have that range be as small as possible. If we consider μ as being a value along a scale that extends infinitely in both directions, we can be 100% sure that μ lies somewhere within the range $+\infty$ and $-\infty$. If we narrow this range, we cannot be certain that the true value of μ lies either within or without the range of values that we have selected. We are no longer 100% confident of our findings.

95% CONFIDENCE INTERVAL

Using our knowledge of a normal distribution, we can narrow this range without too much loss of certainty. There is a 95% chance that the true sample mean will lie within $2s_{\bar{x}}$ units on either side of $\bar{x}$. On average, 19 times out of 20 the unknown μ will be spanned by this interval. The interval or range that we select as boundaries to enclose the value of $\bar{x}$ along a scale with a certain degree of certainty is called the **confidence interval** for the mean. We can use the results obtained from one randomly drawn sample to determine this interval. The boundaries or endpoints of the interval, $\bar{x} - 2s_{\bar{x}}$ and $\bar{x} + 2s_{\bar{x}}$ are called **confidence** limits.

Problem 3:

If the mean OHI-S score for a sample of 400 men in the United States is 1.16 and the variance is .64, what is the 95% confidence interval for μ? What are the confidence limits?

Your Solution:

Similarly, a 99.74%% confidence interval would be expressed as $\bar{x} \pm 3s_{\bar{x}}$. We can select any desired level of confidence as long as it is labeled correctly. Sometimes $\bar{x}$ is stated along with its estimated standard error, $s_{\bar{x}}$, so that the reader can determine what he or she feels is an appropriate confidence interval.

Problem 4:

If the average simplified calculus index for a sample of 625 people in the United States aged 6-74 years is .35 and the standard error is .02, what are the 68.3% confidence limits for μ? The 99.74% confidence limits?

Your Solution:

In chapter 14, the appropriate confidence interval for small sample sizes ($n < 30$) will be discussed. Instead of $\bar{x} \pm 2s_{\bar{x}}$, the 95% confidence interval is determined by $\bar{x} \pm t\, s_{\bar{x}}$. The value for t (with n-1 "degrees of freedom") is slightly larger than 2 and makes our estimation more accurate for smaller samples. It is based on a "t-distribution" which is similar to the normal distribution.

REVIEW

1) A population can be described by its mean, μ, and its variance, σ^2 (or standard deviation σ).

2) A sample from a population can be described by its sample mean, $\bar{x}$, and its sample variance, s^2 (or sample standard deviation, s).

3) Estimated standard error of the sample mean = S.E. = $s_{\bar{x}}$ = $\sqrt{(s^2/n)} = s/\sqrt{n}$.

4) According to the central limit theorem, a group of sample means from samples of size n tend to be shaped like a normal distribution with a mean the same as the population mean, μ, and variance σ^2/n where σ^2 is the true population variance. For fairly large sample sizes ($n \geqslant 30$) the true variance σ^2/n of the sample means may be approximated by the variance of the sample means = s^2/n.

5) The value of μ can be estimated by using confidence intervals or confidence limits. When $n \geqslant 30$:
the 95% confidence interval = $\bar{x} \pm 2s_{\bar{x}}$.
the 95% confidence limits = $\bar{x} - 2s_{\bar{x}}$ and $\bar{x} + 2s_{\bar{x}}$

SOLUTIONS

Problem 1:
The mean OHI-S scores of the 25 random samples from the Boston, Massachusetts population will tend to be normally distributed.

Problem 2:
Variance of one sample, s^2 = .36.
Estimated variance of sample means, s^2/n = .36/400 = .0009
S.E. = $\sqrt{(s^2/n)} = \sqrt{.0009}$ = .03
This can also be calculated as: $s/\sqrt{n}$ = .6/$\sqrt{400}$ = .6/20 = .03

Problem 3:
$\bar{x}$ = 1.16, n = 400, s^2 = .64, s = .8
$s_{\bar{x}} = s/\sqrt{n}$ = .8/$\sqrt{400}$ = .8/20 = .04
95% confidence interval = $\bar{x} \pm 2s_{\bar{x}}$ = 1.16 ± .08
The 95% confidence limits are 1.08 and 1.24.

Problem 4:
$\bar{x}$ = .35, $s_{\bar{x}}$ = .02
68.3% confidence limits = $\bar{x} - s_{\bar{x}}$, $\bar{x} + s_{\bar{x}}$ =
.35 - .02, .35 + .02 = .33, .37
99.74% confidence limits = $\bar{x} - 3s_{\bar{x}}$, $\bar{x} + 3s_{\bar{x}}$ =
.35 - 3(.02), .35 + 3(.02) = .29, .41

POSTTEST 10

A survey was conducted among people who needed at least one tooth extracted to determine the average number of teeth to be extracted and reason for extraction. A sample of 625 adults aged 45-64 years had a mean number of 6.6 teeth needing extraction because of periodontal disease. The sample variance is 196.

Express your estimate for the population mean in terms of a 95% confidence interval.

YOUR ANSWERS
TO POSTTEST 10

Name:

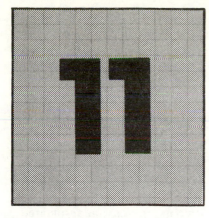

CHAPTER 11

HYPOTHESIS TESTING, SIGNIFICANCE LEVEL AND POWER

INTRODUCTION

In this chapter you will be introduced to the concepts of **hypothesis testing** and **significance level.** When reading the dental literature you will encounter terms such as "null hypothesis," "alternative hypothesis," and "level of significance." For example, you will run across statements like "there was a significant difference between group A and group B ($p < .05$)," or "the difference in rates was significant at the 5% level."

Some statistical theory is applied in making such statements. In order to apply this theory a null hypothesis, alternative hypothesis, and a significance level have been formulated. We will now take a close look at what these terms really mean.

OBJECTIVES

1) You will be able to formulate a null hypothesis and alternative hypothesis in a given experimental situation.
2) You will be able to interpret the level of significance in this same example.
3) You will be able to discuss the concept of power in an experimental situation and know why it is important in determining the size of a sample for that experiment.

FORMULATING A NULL HYPOTHESIS

What is a null hypothesis?

Suppose a study is being conducted to answer questions about differences between two types of pit and fissure sealants. One question that could be asked is, "After ten years, is there a difference in retention between a cold-curing sealant and a sealant that requires ultraviolet light for polymerization?" In this situation, the **null hypothesis** may be stated, "There is no difference between the retention of the two sealants after 10 years." A null hypothesis is usually a statement that **there is no difference between groups** or that one factor is *not* dependent on another (thus it is called *null*).

Problem 1:

Let's try another example. Suppose you wanted to know if one brand of toothpaste, Glow, was better than another brand, Target, in preventing dental caries. What would be the statement of a null hypothesis in this case?

Your Solution:

It may be evident by the previous two examples that associated with the null hypothesis there is always another hypothesis or implied statement concerning the true nature of the problem. This statement is called the **alternative hypothesis.** For our first example, the alternative hypothesis would be, "There *is* a difference between the retention of the two different sealants after 10 years." You can see that a null hypothesis is usually a statement that there is no difference between two or more factors, and the alternative hypothesis is a statement that **some kind of difference exists** and often gives the direction of this relationship.

Problem 2:

Suppose you were interested in setting up null and alternative hypotheses to answer the question, "Does aspirin offer as much post-extraction pain relief for patients as an aspirin with codeine compound?" What would you write as a statement of the alternative hypothesis in this case?

Your Solution:

INVESTIGATING CREDIBILITY OF THE NULL HYPOTHESIS

A **test of a hypothesis** can be thought of as an **investigation of the credibility of the null hypothesis.** The results we obtain of all possibilities from a suitable sample (see chapter 8) are compared with "what we would expect to occur" if the null hypothesis were true. Since sampling variation exists, we can never be absolutely sure that our sample was not unrepresentative of the total population. That is, there is some chance that we might draw a sample which would indicate that the null hypothesis is false when it is really true. The phrase "what we would expect to occur" may seem vague to you at this point. There are mathematical methods for quantifying our "expectation" of what the null hypothesis will produce if it is true. In later chapters we'll look at these mathematical formulae.

SIGNIFICANCE

Suppose a study was conducted in Boston which revealed that 38% of the general practitioners surveyed were in favor of mandatory continuing education requirements for relicensure and 62% were opposed. If this survey had included every single general dentist in Boston, we would be able to say definitely that the null hypothesis (there is no difference between the number of general dentists in Boston who are in favor and who are opposed to mandatory continuing education) is false. However, since we have only the results for a *sample* of dentists, our observed results could be due to chance variation alone.

This is where **significance level** gets into the picture. We know that based on a sample we will always have some chance (or probability) of drawing an unrepresentative sample. Thus, since there is always going to be some chance that the sample is unrepresentative, there is a risk involved in saying the null hypothesis is false when it is really true, based on our sample measurements. The significance level is the **risk we're willing to take that a sample which showed a difference was "misleading."** That is, misleading in the sense that the observed difference was due to chance alone.

For instance the statement, "The difference between the percentage of dentists in favor of and opposed to mandatory continuing education was significant at the 5% level," means that there is a 5% chance that a sample would have shown a difference even if there was no real difference between the two percentages. The "level" is the amount of risk we're willing to take of getting an unrepresentative sample. Another way of stating this result is, "Only one sample out of 20 (1/20 = .05 or 5%) would show as great a difference as this sample did if the null hypothesis were true." Under these conditions we conclude that the null hypothesis statement is false, knowing that there is a 1 in 20 chance that we were fooled by a misleading sample. Concluding the null hypothesis is false at the 5% level can be thought of as *reasonable evidence* against the null hypothesis. Concluding the null hypothesis is false at the 1% level can be thought of as *strong evidence* against the null hypothesis.

Problem 3:

Let's try an example concerning significance. Does *5% level of significance* mean,

1) We're taking a 5% risk of miswriting the null hypothesis?
2) We're taking a 5% risk that our sample is unrepresentative if the null hypothesis is true?
3) We're taking a 5% risk of getting an unrepresentative sample if the alternative hypothesis is true?
4) We're taking a 5% risk of making a wrong decision, regardless of which hypothesis is true?

Your Solution:

In journals you will find significance levels expressed as $p < 0.05$ or $p < 0.01$. The statement $p < 0.05$ means that there is less than a 5% risk that our sample is a misrepresentative sample if the null hypothesis is true. This would be reasonable evidence for concluding that the null hypothesis is false.

Problem 4:
What do you think the statement $p < 0.01$ means?

Your Solution:

Another notation that is used in journals is often *N.S. or S,* referring to *non-significant or significant* results. Sometimes asterisks are used, **, **, **** referring to significance at the *5%, 1% and 0.1%* levels, respectively. However, it is recommended that the actual p- values that the researcher obtained be reported so that the reader can decide whether or not to *accept or reject* the null hypothesis. It must be kept in mind that a large difference between two study variables may not appear to be significant if a sample size is small and that small differences between two study variables may appear significant if the sample size is large.

FURTHER INVESTIGATION OF THE NULL HYPOTHESIS

If the aim of a study is to determine whether or not to reject the null hypothesis, how can we be sure that we are making the right decision? Suppose we go back to the example where the null hypothesis states, "There is no difference between the amount of post-extraction pain relief experienced between patients given aspirin and those given aspirin with codeine." The alternative hypothesis is, of course, that there is a difference. If we wanted to make the right decision we would

1) reject the null hypothesis when the treatments are different or
2) not reject the null hypothesis when indeed the treatments do not differ.

Remember, when we discussed significance levels, we were assuming that the null hypothesis is true; in other words, there really is no difference in pain relief between aspirin and aspirin with codeine. With a significance level at 5% under the null hypothesis 95% of the time we will get a sample that shows no difference between the two treatments. In addition, we take only a 5% risk of obtaining a sample that shows a significant difference between the two treatments. In other words, we only have a 5% chance of making a wrong decision:

we would mistakenly reject the null 5% of the time, when indeed the null is true. This type of wrong decision is known as a Type I or alpha (α) error. A randomly selected representative sample (see chapter 8) helps to avoid making an alpha error.

What happens if in reality the treatments do differ? In other words, if the alternative hypothesis is true, post-extraction pain relief treatment with aspirin versus aspirin with codeine are different. There is a chance, of course, that we will make a wrong decision in this case as well: we'll declare there is no difference between aspirin and aspirin with codeine when in fact there is a difference. This type of error is known as a Type II or beta (β) error. How can we insure that we do not make an error, but instead we reject the null when the alternative hypothesis is true?

Power:

The ability of a study to detect a difference between treatments if the alternative hypothesis is true is known as the power of a study. Power is dependent upon 1) the magnitude of difference between the two treatments to be detected 2) the number of study subjects in each treatment group, 3) the population variance and 4) the α error we are using.

Identifying the difference between two treatment groups that is to be detected and in turn, determining the number of subjects needed before the study begins will help in avoiding a beta error. To do this, the true difference between treatment groups and the population variance must be guessed or estimated, from previous work if available. It is important to "guess" as accurately as possible, because the beta error is very sensitive to the quantities. Determination of the sample size is, therefore, dependent upon 1) what level of α and β errors you as an investigator are willing to risk. 2) the magnitude of treatment difference to be detected, and 3) the underlying population variance.

To illustrate how both the sample size and the differences between treatment groups affect our chances of making a beta error, let's take the earlier example where we wanted to know if the toothpaste, Glow, was better than the toothpaste, Target, in preventing dental caries. Our null hypothesis stated there was no difference in cariostatic effect of the two toothpastes while the alternative states that Target is better than Glow. Let's assume we want:

1) to be 95% sure that we do not reject the null hypothesis when the null is true. In other words, we are only willing to risk a 5% chance of making an alpha error (α).

2) We also want to be 90% sure we will reject the null when the alternative is true (Power = .90).

Because the beta error is the complement of power, they are mathematically related as follows:

$$\beta = 1 - \text{Power}$$

Thus, if Power equals 90%, this means we are only willing to risk a 10% chance of making a beta error ($\beta = .10$). Depending upon the suspected difference that Target is better than Glow, the required sample size will vary. Again, let's assume we suspect that the subjects who received Glow will have a 25% improvement in their caries experience whereas Target users will improve 50% (in other words, another 25% beyond the Glow users). Table 11.1 shows the minimum sample sizes per treatment group required to insure against making a beta error when alpha has been set at .05 and beta has been set at .10. By looking at the table we find that we need at least 77 subjects in each treatment group to insure with 90% probability that we even have the ability to detect a 25% difference between the effects of the two toothpastes. It should also be noted that if the α error is increased, then the β error is reduced for an experiment with a given sample size.

Table 11.1

SAMPLE SIZE REQUIRED PER TREATMENT GROUP
Assuming $\alpha = .05$ and $\beta = .10$

Success Rate for Worse Treatment (Glow)	Improvement in Success Rate with the Better Treatment (Target)			
	5%	10%	25%	35%
10%	910	260	54	31
25%	1680	440	77	40
50%	2100	520	77	35

Source: Levenstein, MJ and Bishop, YMM. "Analysis and Reporting as Causes of Controversies." In: Rosenor, VM and Rothchild, M (eds.) *Controversies in Clinical Care*. New York, Spectrum, 1981.

Problem 5:
What happens to the required sample size if we should overestimate the difference between Glow and Target (if, for instance, the difference between the two toothpastes is really 10% and not 25% as we originally assumed)?

Your Solution:

Problem 6:
Assuming a Type I error of 5% and a power of 90%, what sample size would be required if Glow results in a 25% reduction in dental caries and Target results in a 30% reduction in dental caries?

Your Solution:

From these last examples we can see that the smaller the difference to be detected the more subjects we will need to be able to make the right decision. Also, if we are willing to accept a higher risk of making a Type II error, we can get away with using a smaller sample size. Alternatively, if we wish to decrease the chance of making a Type II error, we do so at the risk of increasing a Type I error. Clearly, an investigator has to wonder why a study should even be done if the sample size is inadequate to detect the true difference between treatments. However, because of the cost and time involved in using more study subjects, an investigator must weigh the trade-offs: we want to keep the number of study subjects down, yet still maintain the study's power. A study which can pull off such a balancing act is referred to as being efficient. Ideally, the closer we can guess the difference, the better our choice of sample size will be, resulting in a more powerful and efficient study.

It should be clear now that a large difference between two study variables may not appear to be significant if a sample size is too small. Interestingly, if a sample size is too large a small difference between two study variables may appear "very significant." This phenomenon becomes clear from Table 1; suppose 2100 subjects use either Glow or Target and Glow users experience a 50% improvement in their experiences with caries whereas Target users experience a 55% improvement. This 5% difference between the two groups would be "statistically significant." However, it's up to the thoughtful investigator (or clinician) to determine if that small difference is clinically significant.

REVIEW

1) A **null hypothesis** is a statement that there is no difference between two or more treatments or factors under investigation.
2) An **alternative hypothesis** is a statement that there is a difference between two or more treatments or factors under investigation, and can indicate the direction of the difference.
3) After formulation of the null and alternative hypotheses, a study sample is selected to "test the credibility of the hypothesis." Do the results of our sample represent reality? By selecting a **level of significance,** we choose the amount of risk we are willing to take that our sample is representative. A 5% significance level indicates we have a 95% chance that our sample is representative.
4) Performing a significance test on the data obtained from our sample provides us with a value from which to judge whether to reject the null hypothesis. If the significance level is set at 5%, and the value from our significance test is $p < .05$ we can then reject our null hypothesis.
5) From the results of the significance test, we can make four different decisions about the null hypothesis. The aim of a study is to make the right decision.

Table 11.2

Result of significance test	Null hypothesis is true	Alternative hypothesis is true
Statistically significant, therefore reject null hypothesis	Type I error or α (alpha) error	correct decision
Not statistically significant, therefore do not reject null hypothesis	correct decision	Type II error or β (beta) error

6) **Type I (or alpha) error.** This wrong decision is a result of rejecting the null hypothesis when in reality the null is true. Setting the significance level at 5% connotes that, as a researcher, you are willing to take a 5% chance of making an alpha error.

7) A randomly selected representative sample and a good study design help to improve the probability of avoiding an alpha error.

8) **Type II (or beta) error.** This wrong decision is a result of failing to reject the null hypothesis when in reality the null is not true.

9) The **power** of a study is the chance of detecting the difference between two samples if the alternative hypothesis is true. By increasing the power of a study, we can decrease our risk of making a beta error (beta = 1 - Power).

10) Power is dependent upon 1) the magnitude of the difference to be detected, 2) the study sample size, and 3) the α error. If the difference is large, fewer sample subjects are needed. Conversely, if the difference is small, a large sample size is needed. Moreover, if the α error is allowed to increase, β error will decrease.

SOLUTIONS

Problem 1:

If you said something like, "There is *no* difference between the cariostatic effect of Glow and Target," then you've got the idea.

Problem 2:

If you said, "There is a difference in the amount of post-extraction pain relief experienced between patients given aspirin and those given aspirin with codeine," you've got the basic idea of an alternative hypothesis.

Problem 3:

Statement 2 is correct. Remember, the 5% means: 1) We assume the null hypothesis is true; 2) If this assumption is correct, there is a 5% chance we'll get a misleading sample.

Problem 4:

There is a 1% risk that our sample is misrepresentative if the null hypothesis is true.

This would be regarded as strong evidence for accepting the alternative hypothesis.

Problem 5:

If we should overestimate the difference between Glow and Target our sample size will be too small to detect a difference and thus, there is a good chance we would not reject the null hypothesis, and instead, assume they were equally effective in preventing caries when in fact Target is better - that is, we'll make a beta or Type II error. For instance if Target is only 10% better than Glow, we would need 440 subjects per treatment group, not the 77 we had originally planned.

Problem 6:

Reading from Table 11.1, a sample size of 1,680 individuals per treatment group would be required.

POSTTEST 11

When you read a statement which gives the results of a comparison in terms of a significance level or a percentage of significance, there are three concepts asociated with that statement, the null hypothesis, the alternative hypothesis, and level of significance. Let's try to combine these three concepts.

Suppose after taking measurements of periodontal pocket depth for two groups of patients, the result is stated, "There was a significant difference in the average periodontal pocket depth between group A and group B, at the 5% level."

1) Which of the following is a suitable statement of the null hypothesis?
   a) There is a difference in the average periodontal pocket depth between individuals in group A and group B.
   b) There is no difference in the average periodontal pocket depth between individuals in group A and group B.
   c) There is no difference in sampling variation between groups A and B.
   d) Group A and group B have different types of individuals with respect to the periodontal pocket depth.

2) Is one of these four statements a suitable formulation of the alternative hypothesis? If yes, which one? If no, what is the alternative hypothesis?

3) Now, what about the level of significance? Did the author imply:
   a) There is a 5% chance that he observed a difference?
   b) He agrees with the null hypothesis, knowing that there is at most a 5% chance he had a misrepresentative sample?
   c) He disagrees with the null hypothesis, knowing that there is at most a 5% chance he had a misrepresentative sample?
   d) He disagrees with the alternative hypothesis 5% of the time?

4) If we wanted to be more convinced that the author's conclusions were valid, what other information would be useful? Why?
   a) The value of the beta error.
   b) The mean and standard error of Group A and of Group B.
   c) The sample size of each group.
   d) All of the above.

YOUR ANSWERS
TO POSTTEST 11

Name:

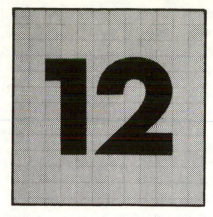

CHAPTER 12

THE CHI-SQUARE STATISTIC APPLIED TO A 2x2 TABLE

INTRODUCTION

You may recall that in the chapter on hypothesis testing, we stated that there are mathematical methods for evaluating the credibility of the null hypothesis. One of these methods is the **chi-square test.** This test is commonly used and can be applied without sophisticated mathematical tools. The symbol χ^2 is named "chi-square" and refers to a statistical distribution on which the test is based. In this chapter we will use this method to look at a specific type of situation. We will look at a problem where we are comparing two groups (say Group A and Group B) with respect to some characteristic. We will have a tabulation of the number of Group A and Group B observations as:

Table 12.1

	With Characteristic	Without Characteristic
Group A		
Group B		

Our null hypothesis is "there is no difference between the proportion of those in Group A with the characteristic and the proportion of those in Group B with the characteristic." In this chapter you will see how we can make a calculation to investigate this null hypothesis quantitatively.

OBJECTIVES

1) Given a statement of the results of a clinical experiment, you will be able to construct a 2x2 table and calculate a chi-square statistic.
2) You will be able to interpret for this clinical experiment the calculated value of a chi-square statistic.
3) You will be able to identify from four possible choices a correct interpretation of a chi-square statistic.

2 x 2 TABLE

Suppose you were conducting a study to compare the post-operative sequelae experienced by patients receiving single visit and multiple visit endodontic treatment on teeth which had received the same diagnosis. After completing treatment, the patients were asked to return postcards which indicated whether or not they had any post-operative pain. The following table shows the results:

Table 12.2

	With Characteristic Pain	Without Characteristic No Pain	Total
Group A: Single Visit	50	32	82
Group B: Multiple Visit	75	133	208

This table can be seen to be of a similar form to that indicated in the introduction. The table tells us that there were 82 patients who were treated in a single visit and 208 patients who received a multivisit procedure (a total of 290 patients in both groups). You can see that there are two groups and two characteristics. This type of table is known as a **2 by 2 table.** The "by" is symbolized by an "x," and we write 2x2. In fact, there are 2x2 = 4 categories of observations in the table: single visit patients with pain, single visit patients without pain, multivisit patients with pain, and multivisit patients without pain.

Problem 1:
Looking at the table, how many of the patients in the combined sample of the two different groups experienced pain?

Your Solution:

Our complete table now is:

Table 12.3

	Pain	No Pain	Total
Single Visit	50	32	82
Multiple Visit	75	133	208
Total (both groups)	125	165	290

Remember, this is still a 2x2 table; the totals are not a separate group or characteristic.

USING THE TABLE TO EVALUATE A NULL HYPOTHESIS

We're now ready to take the information in the table to evaluate an appropriate null hypothesis. (Remember that the null hypothesis was established *before* the study was conducted.)

Problem 2:

Applying the definition in the chapter on hypothesis testing, what was the null hypothesis in this example?

Your Solution:

Now, if that null hypothesis is true, then there should be no difference between the proportion of single visit patients who experienced pain and the proportion of both treatment groups combined who experienced pain. (The same holds true for multiple visit patients.) Does this point make sense?

Let's do some calculations to illustrate it further.

Problem 3:

What is the proportion of patients (both groups combined) who reported post-operative pain in this sample?

Your Solution:

Now if there is really *no* difference in the proportion of patients reporting pain between the two groups (single and multivisit), *each* group should have approximately the same proportion of patients reporting pain or .431.

Assume that the proportion of patients reporting pain for both groups combined was equal to .431, and you knew that there were 49 patients sampled. If the null hypothesis is true (no difference in proportion between groups), how many of those 49 patients would you expect to experience post-operative pain? You would expect there to be 49 x .431 = 21 patients who experience post-operative pain.

Problem 4:

Looking at the table, how many multiple visit patients would you expect to experience pain if the null hypothesis is true?

Your Solution:

In the same way we can calculate the expected number of patients in each treatment group who did not report any pain. The expected number of single visit patients who did not report any pain = 82 x .569 = 47, and the expected number of multivisit patients who did not report any pain = 208 x .569 = 118.

Remember that by "expected" we mean the number in each group we anticipate seeing if the null hypothesis is true, i.e., if there is no difference between the two treatment groups with regard to post-operative pain.

The **chi-square statistic** can be thought of in general terms as a quantitative comparison between what we calculated as *expected* (based on the proportion of the characteristic for both groups combined) and what we actually *observed*. Let's summarize what we calculated as expected numbers for each category and what was actually observed in the table.

Table 12.4

Category	Observed	Expected
Single visit: Pain	50	35
Single visit: No pain	32	47
Multiple visit: pain	75	90
Multiple visit: no pain	133	118

An easy way of calculating the expected value for each of the four cells in the 2x2 table is by using the following formula:

$$\text{Expected value} = \frac{\text{Row total} \times \text{Column total}}{\text{Grand total}}$$

For the cell, "Single Visit with Pain," the computation is:

$$(82 \cdot 125)/290 = 35$$

If the null hypothesis is true, the difference between observed and expected should be small. The larger these differences are, the less credible is the null hypothesis. The chi-square statistic is based on this fact. To begin computing the chi-square statistic, we look at each category and

1) Compute the difference between observed (O) and expected (E) values (O-E).
2) Square that difference, $(O-E)^2$.
3) Divide the squared difference by the expected value, $(O-E)^2/E$.

Let's take an example from our table. For the category "Multiple Visits, Pain."

1) The difference between observed and expected is 75 - 90 = -15.
2) The square of the difference is $(-15)^2 = 225$.
3) The squared difference divided by the expected number in this category is 225/90 = 2.50.

Problem 5:

Try steps 1, 2, and 3 for the category "Multiple Visits, No Pain." What would be the squared difference divided by the expected number?

Your Solution:

Our final step is to sum the values of step 3 over all categories. The final result we obtain is the value of the chi-square statistic. It is useful to do the computation using the following table, where the *observed* number in each category is denoted by an "O" and the *expected* number by "E."

Table 12.5

Category	O	E	(O − E)	$(O - E)^2$	$(O - E)^2/E$
1					
2					
3					
4					
Total					

The total in the last column is the value of the chi-square statistic.

One value of this table is its use as a mechanism for checking your calculations. The expected numbers we calculated earlier can be thought of as a reallocation of the total number of observations in the table. That is, to calculate expected values, we started with the total number of observations and worked backwards. Thus, the sum of all expected values will be equal to the sum of all observed values (i.e., the E column total = the O column total). There might be a slight difference between the totals due to rounding off error, but any large difference indicates a calculation error.

Problem 6:

What about the O-E total? Since the totals for O and E are equal, the cell expected numbers cannot be consistently larger or smaller than the observed values. Therefore, O-E cannot be consistently positive or negative. Positive values for O-E in some cells will be balanced off by negative values in other cells. What would you expect the O-E total to be?

Your Solution:

Problem 7:

Recall that there are four categories in our example, one for each cell in the 2x2 table. What is the chi-square statistic for this table?

Your Solution:

INTERPRETING THE CHI-SQUARE STATISTIC

Remember we said if the null hypothesis is true, the difference O-E for each category (or cell) should be small, and thus the chi-square value should be small. Of course, if the null hypothesis is false, the chi-square statistic calculation will be larger. So if we observe a very small value of chi-square, we would tend to accept the null hypothesis (i.e., there is no difference between groups), and if we observe a very large value of chi-square, we would tend to reject the null hypothesis (i.e., there is a difference between groups). Notice, however, that this line of reasoning with its statistical support never really *proves* anything. We are still faced with a decision to accept or reject something in a state of uncertainty, only now we have limited the chances of making a mistake and made it a relatively small chance.

At this point you may be asking, "How small is small?" or "Above what value of the chi-square statistic do we reject the null hypothesis?" Well, remember that there is always a possibility that a large value of chi-square could be observed by chance alone. Statisticians have tabulated the probabilities of chi-square being above certain values when the null hypothesis is really true. These values are called **"critical values."** They are computed to correspond to the significance level of the test (recall from chapter 11 that the concept of significance level is the probability of getting a unrepresentative sample when the null hypothesis is true). For example, for a 2x2 table the probability that the chi-square statistic is greater than 3.84 when the null hypothesis is true is (.05). Thus, for a test of hypothesis at the 5% level, 3.84 is the critical value. *(Note: the use of degrees of freedom, which is necessary to determine the critical value, is taken up in the next chapter.)* We say the null hypothesis is probably false, that is, we reject the null hypothesis, if we observe a chi-square value 3.84 or larger. Otherwise we do not reject the null hypothesis - we do not find a significant difference.

SUMMARY

If the chi-square statistic is *equal to or larger than* the critical value that we have selected:

1) We have found a significant difference between groups.
2) This difference is unlikely to be due to random process or chance alone, and
3) We *reject* the null hypothesis.

If the chi-square statistic is *smaller* than the critical value that we have selected:

1) We have found a nonsignificant difference between groups in this sample.
2) The results obtained may be due to chance or sampling variation and thus are inconclusive, and
3) We *accept* or *fail to reject* the null hypothesis.

Again, this does not mean that we have proved the null hypothesis, only that we do not have sufficient evidence from this particular experiment to contradict it.

Problem 8:

Looking back at our example, if the significance level of the test of hypothesis was 5%, would we reject the null hypothesis (in other words, find a significant difference between the proportion of patients who were treated in one visit and experienced pain and those who experienced pain after several visits) or fail to reject it, based on the calculated chi-square statistic?

Your Solution:

Problem 9:

Suppose the chi-square statistic had been calculated as 2.71. Now, what would we say about the null hypothesis?

Your Solution:

REVIEW

1) The chi-square statistic is the sum of the values

$$\Sigma \; \frac{(\text{Observed - Expected})^2}{\text{Expected}} = \Sigma \; \frac{(O\text{-}E)^2}{E}$$

where $(O\text{-}E)^2/E$ is calculated for each category or cell in the table.

2) The chi-square value thus calculated is compared with a tabulated critical value to determine whether we accept or reject the null hypothesis.

SOLUTIONS

Problem 1:

There are 50 + 75 = 125 patients that experienced post-operative pain.

Problem 2:

You should have said something like, "There is no difference between the proportion of patients experiencing post-operative pain after a single visit endodontic procedure and the proportion experiencing pain after a multiple visit procedure." We brought this up because it's important to remember that the purpose of applying the chi-square statistic is to evaluate the credibility of this statement based on the data.

Problem 3:

Looking at the table, we see that there were 125 patients reporting pain and 290 total, so the proportion is 125/290 = .431.

Problem 4:

Did you calculate 208 x .431 = 90? That's right. There are 208 multiple visit patients in the sample, so if there's no difference in proportion between patients in the two treatment groups, we should expect the number of multiple visit patients who experience post-operative pain = (total number of multivisit patients in sample) x (proportion of both groups combined who experienced pain) = 208 x .431 = 90.

Problem 5:

If you said *1.91*, you're on the track. The 1.91 was computed by $(133\text{-}118)^2/118 = 1.91$, using steps 1, 2 and 3.

Problem 6:

Did you say *zero*? That's correct. Note that we have two methods for checking calculations. First, the O column total should equal the E column total. Second, the O-E total should be zero.

Problem 7:

Did you get 15.63 as the chi-square value? The calculation of this number was accomplished as follows:

Table 12.6

Category	O	E	(O − E)	$(O − E)^2$	$(O − E)^2/E$
1	50	35	15	225	$225/35 = 6.43$
2	32	47	−15	225	$225/47 = 4.79$
3	75	90	−15	225	$225/90 = 2.50$
4	133	118	15	225	$225/118 = 1.91$
Total	290	290	0	—	15.63

The chi-square value is the total of the last column equal to 15.63.

Problem 8:

We would reject the null hypothesis. The observed chi-square value of 15.63 is greater than 3.84, the critical value for a 5% level test.

Problem 9:

Did you say, "We would accept the null hypothesis" or "We would not find a significant difference?" Either of these statements is correct. The value of 2.71 is less than the critical value of 3.84 and thus we accept the null hypothesis. Note once again that we have not proved it, rather we just do not have sufficient evidence to the contrary.

POST TEST 12

In the same endodontic study, 250 patients were later re-examined radiographically for evidence of osseous healing. There were 76 who had been treated in a single visit and 174 who had been treated in multiple visits. Of those treated during a single visit, 65 showed evidence of osseous healing; of the patients who were treated in multiple visits, 18 did not show evidence of healing by radiographic examination.

1) Construct a 2x2 table for the two treatment groups showing the number in each group who were healing and non-healing.
2) Calculate the expected number of patients with evidence of healing and non-healing for each group, based on the table above.
3) Calculate the value of the chi-square statistic for this table.
4) Select the answer which best completes the following statement. A chi-square statistic is a value which:
   a) Gives us a measure of how well we construct the 2x2 table.
   b) Gives us a measure of the level of significance of the test.
   c) Is compared with a critical value to establish the level of significance.
   d) Is compared with a critical value to determine whether we accept or reject the null hypothesis.
5) Test the null hypothesis of no difference in healing between the two treatment groups at the 5% level. The chi-square critical value for this case is 3.84.

YOUR ANSWERS TO POSTTEST 12

Name:

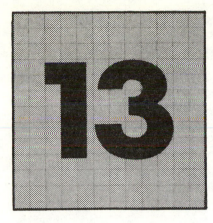

CHAPTER 13

RXC TABLES AND DEGREES OF FREEDOM

INTRODUCTION

The previous chapter has introduced some of the basic principles you need to be able to analyze tables of data with more than just two rows and two columns. In general we say that a table with r rows and c columns is an rxc table, also referred to as a contingency table. However, one new idea must be introduced before you can proceed with larger tables, and that is the concept of degrees of freedom. You will then be able to analyze a table of any size in much the same way as you did the 2x2 table.

OBJECTIVES

1) You will be able to calculate the number of degrees of freedom of the chi-square statistic to investigate the null hypothesis of no association between the row and column variables for any rxc table.
2) You will be able to calculate the value of the chi-square statistic for any rxc table.
3) Using a table of the chi-square distribution (Table 13.5), you will be able to determine the appropriate value with which the calculated chi-square statistic must be compared in order to assess the credibility of the null hypothesis.
4) You will be able to interpret the chi-square statistic calculated in fulfilling Objective 2.

DEGREES OF FREEDOM

Suppose that you are analyzing the results of a survey that was undertaken to determine the relationship between attitude toward fluoridation and knowledge of fluoridation. The respondents were chosen to be a representative cross-section of the general public. The results for this particular question are summarized in Table 13.1. This table has 3 rows and 3 columns.

You will notice that the row and column totals are included in the table. Consider these totals to be fixed quantities and the cells inside the table to be variable. The first problem introduces the concept of **degrees of freedom.**

Table 13.1

NUMBER OF RESPONDENTS BY ATTITUDE TOWARD FLUORIDATION AND KNOWLEDGE OF FLUORIDATION

Attitude toward Fluoridation	Knowledge of Fluoridation			
	Correct	Uncertain	Incorrect	Total
Favorable	209	80	151	440
Undecided	61	67	31	159
Unfavorable	32	25	20	77
Total	302	172	202	676

Source: Adapted from Metz, Stafford A., An Analysis of Some Determinants of Attitude Toward Flouridation. *Social Forces,* Vol. 44, June 1966, p. 477-484

Problem 1:

Assume that you were given only the total fixed values for the rows and columns in Table 13.1 and the 9 inner cells were empty. How many of these 9 cells could be filled in with any numerical value, without restrictions from the other cells? (You may find this problem a little difficult. Think carefully.)

Your Solution:

The first two cells of the first and second rows can be filled in without restriction, but then all remaining cells are determined by subtraction from the fixed row and column totals. Think of the third row and third column cells as buffers. Hence, this table has 4 degrees of freedom, as only four cells can be given numerical values *freely*.

In general an rxc table has (r-1) x (c-1) degrees of freedom. To check this for the 3x3 table we see that (3-1) x (3-1) = 4.

CALCULATION OF THE CHI-SQUARE STATISTIC

The main point of interest in this table is whether there are any differences between people's knowledge of fluoridation and their attitude toward fluoridation.

The null hypothesis may be stated as follows: There are no differences between those who answered the knowledge question about fluoridation correctly, incorrectly or were uncertain about the answer, and how they feel about fluoridating public water supplies.

Now if the null hypothesis were true, we would expect the proportion of those with correct knowledge of fluoridation who favor fluoridation to be nearly the same as the proportion of those with incorrect knowledge or uncertain knowledge who favor fluoridation. We see that overall 65.1% (440/676 x 100) of the respondents in this sample were in favor of fluoridation. Hence, if we believe the null hypothesis, we would expect about 65.1% of each "knowledge" group to feel this way. We may calculate what we expect in each cell as we did for the 2x2 table. In the first cell, we would expect 65.1% of 302, or 196.6; in the second cell, 65.1% of 172, or 112.0, and so on.

The following formula which is used to calculate the expected value of a particular cell in an rxc table is the same formula that was used in chapter 12 for a 2x2 table.

$$\frac{\text{Row total} \times \text{Column total}}{\text{Grand Total}}$$

Now we can proceed to calculate the value of the chi-square statistic for our 3x3 table. The arithmetic manipulations are similar to those for the 2x2 table in the previous chapter.

Table 13.2 summarizes the procedures involved. The 9 cells in the 3x3 table have each been assigned a number, starting from the top left hand corner and moving from left to right to the bottom right hand corner. The assigned numbers, 1-9, appear under the column "category."

Table 13.2

CALCULATION OF CHI-SQUARE STATISTIC FOR 3 x 3 TABLE

Category	O	E	O – E	$(O - E)^2$	$(O - E)^2/E$
1	209	196.6	12.4	153.76	.78
2	80	112.0	–32.0	1,024.00	9.14
3	151	131.5	19.5	380.25	2.89
4	61	71.0	–10.0	100.00	1.41
5	67	40.5	26.5	702.25	17.34
6	31	47.5	–16.5	272.25	5.73
7	32	34.4	–2.4	5.76	.17
8	25	19.6	5.4	29.16	1.49
9	20	23.0	–3.0	9.00	.39
	676	676-1	-0.1		39.34

The "O" or *observed* column may then be completed by reference to the table being analyzed. The "E" or *expected* column follows by multiplying the appropriate row and column totals and dividing by the grand total. For example, category 5 refers to the cell in the second row and second column. The expected value for this cell under the null hypothesis is:

$$\frac{\text{Second row total} \times \text{Second column total}}{\text{Grand total}}$$

or in this case is $(159 \times 172)/676 = 40.5$.

As a check on all the "E" values, add the entries in that column. The total of expected values should be the same as the total of the observed values, allowing for rounding errors.

The "O-E" column follows easily. Again, note that the total of this column should be zero, or close to it. The entries in the "O-E" column are squared in the next column and then divided by "E" to give the contributions to the chi-square value in the final column.

As in the 2x2 table, we sum the final column to get the chi-square value, in this case 39.34. We now use this chi-square value to determine the credibility of the null hypothesis. However, we need to determine the appropriate value from a table of the χ^2 distribution with which to compare our calculated value of 39.34 so as to assess this credibility. The statistical table at the end of this chapter describes the χ^2 distribution and allows us to determine the appropriate comparison values for different tables (i.e., different degrees of freedom) and different levels of significance.

Table 13.1 has 4 degrees of freedom. We enter the χ^2 table at the end of the chapter in the row where DF = 4. The row of entries corresponding to DF = 4 gives numerical levels which must be reached by our calculated chi-square value in order to reject the null hypothesis with a given level of evidence. Recall that in chapter 11 we discussed levels of significance and indicated that the 1% level was strong evidence and the 5% level moderate evidence for rejecting the null hypothesis. Suppose we decide that we need strong evidence for rejecting our null hypothesis that the different knowledge groups have the same attitudes toward fluoridation. Then we move along the row DF = 4 until we get to the 1% column. The value for comparison is 13.277. Hence, if our calculated chi-square value is greater than or equal to 13.277, we have strong evidence to reject the null hypothesis. Our value of 39.29 is much greater than 13.277 and so we would conclude that the 3 different knowledge groups did not have the same attitudes toward fluoridation. Further description of the original data in terms of percentages would describe the differences present in a direct manner.

REVIEW

1) An rxc table has (r-1)(c-1) degrees of freedom.

2) Given an rxc table and a null hypothesis concerning the lack of association between rows and columns that must be investigated, first calculate the expected values for each cell under this null hypothesis. In general:

$$E = \frac{\text{Row total} \times \text{Column total}}{\text{Grand total}}$$

Therefore, for the first cell we calculate:

$$\frac{\text{First row total} \times \text{First column total}}{\text{Grand total}}$$

Then moving left to right in our given table, we calculate:

$$\frac{\text{First row total} \times \text{Second column total}}{\text{Grand total}}$$

3) We go through succeeding rows until we have calculated the *expected* value for all cells in the rxc table, remembering to record each score on the chi-square calculation table:

Table 13.3

Category	O	E	(O – E)	(O – E)^2	(O – E)^2/E
X	X	X	X	X	X
X	X	X	X	X	X

4) The final column total in the calculation table is the chi-square value, which you then compare for significance with the corresponding figure in a distribution table. Remember to enter the table at the correct number of degrees of freedom.

SOLUTIONS

Problem 1:

Did you say *four*? Good. Here's the explanation. The first cell can be filled with any number, say 200 (provided, of course, it is less than 440, the row total). Then the next cell can also be filled without restriction, say 100. However, the row total is constrained to be 440, and so the third cell in that row must be 140 if the first two cells are 200 and 100.

POSTTEST 13

Below on this page you will see Table 13.4 which describes the attitudes toward fluoridation held by people of different income levels who were interviewed in a state-wide health interview survey in Massachusetts in 1980. (Lambert, CA et al. *Risk factors and life style: A statewide health interview survey*. New England Journal of Medicine 306:1048, 1982.)

1) State an appropriate null hypothesis for Table 13.4.
2) Calculate the number of degrees of freedom for Table 13.4.
3) Calculate the value of the chi-square statistic for Table 13.4.
4) Determine the appropriate value with which the chi-square statistic must be compared in order to assess the credibility of the null hypothesis at the 1% and 5% levels of significance.
5) Identify from the following choices, a suitable interpretation of your analysis:
   a) There is strong evidence to reject the null hypothesis.
   b) There is strong evidence to accept the null hypothesis.
   c) There is moderate evidence to accept the null hypothesis.
6) Calculate the number of degrees of freedom for a 5x4 table.
7) What would be the critical chi-square statistic for a 5x4 table to show moderate evidence for rejecting a null hypothesis?

Table 13.4

NUMBER OF RESPONDENTS BY ATTITUDE TOWARD FLUORIDATION AND INCOME			
Attitude Toward Fluoridation	Income		
	<$10,000	$10–20,000	>$20,000	Total
Favor	127	181	271	579
Oppose	48	72	77	197
No Opinion	42	44	36	122
Total	217	297	384	898

5% AND 1% UPPER PERCENTAGE POINTS
OF THE CHI-SQUARE DISTRIBUTION

DF	5%	1%
1	3.8415	6.6349
2	5.9915	9.2103
3	7.8147	11.3449
4	9.4877	13.2767
5	11.0705	15.0863
6	12.5916	16.8119
7	14.0671	18.4753
8	15.5073	20.0902
9	16.9190	21.6660
10	18.3070	23.2092
11	19.6751	24.7250
12	21.0261	26.2170
13	22.3620	27.6882
14	23.6848	29.1412
15	24.9958	30.5779
16	26.2962	31.9999
17	27.5871	33.4087
18	28.8693	34.8053
19	30.1435	36.1909
20	31.4104	37.5662
21	32.6706	38.9322
22	33.9244	40.2894
23	35.1725	41.6384
24	36.4150	42.9798
25	37.6525	44.3141
26	38.8851	45.6417
27	40.1133	46.9629
28	41.3371	48.2782
29	42.5570	49.5879
30	43.7730	50.8922
40	55.7585	63.6907
50	67.5048	76.1539
60	79.0819	88.3794
70	90.5312	100.425
80	101.879	112.329
90	113.145	124.116
100	124.342	135.807

YOUR ANSWERS TO POSTTEST 13

Name:

CHAPTER 14

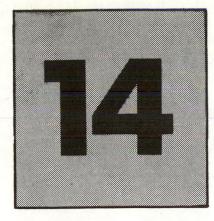

THE t-TEST

INTRODUCTION

In chapter 11, the ideas of hypothesis tests and levels of significance were introduced, and in chapters 12 and 13 the chi-square test was presented for testing certain hypotheses about proportions and percents. Sometimes one wishes to test hypotheses about measurements taken on a *continuous variable*. Often this takes the form of a comparison between two or more treatments, e.g., the effect of two different drugs on blood pressure reduction. We shall discuss here a test that is commonly used for comparing two treatments, which is called the **t-test.**

OBJECTIVES

1) You will be able to formulate one-sided and two-sided hypotheses about the comparison of *two* treatments.
2) You will be able to test these hypotheses at a given level of significance, using either a **two-sample (unpaired) t-test** or a **one-sample (paired) t-test.**
3) In order to use the t-test you will learn to use **t-tables.**

TWO-SAMPLE OR UNPAIRED T-TEST

Suppose a group of 15 people gave informed consent to participate in a study designed to test two new anti-caries vaccines. Seven people received one type of vaccine, called Cariestat, while the remaining eight received the other type, Zerocay. Several days following the injections, samples of their saliva and gingival crevicular fluid were monitored to record levels of a critical immunological component of the vaccine, fluorocal salivarius. *(Note: This is a hypothetical situation with fictitious names!)* Baseline readings of fluorocal salivarius prior to receiving either vaccine was zero since it does not occur naturally in the human body. The amount of fluorocal salivarius found in the saliva samples of the subjects in each test group 3 days after the injections are given in Table 14.1.

We wish to test if the level of fluorocal salivarius found in the saliva differ for the two vaccines. We may state our null hypothesis as:

$$H_0: \mu_C = \mu_Z \text{ vs. the alternative } H_1: \mu_C \neq \mu_Z$$

where μ_C and μ_Z are the mean levels of fluorocal salivarius after treatment with Cariestat and Zerocay respectively. Our null hypothesis states that the two anticaries vaccines produce the same level of the critical component fluorocal salivarius in the saliva, and our alternative states that there is a difference between the effects of the two vaccines in this respect.

Table 14.1

FLUOROCAL SALIVARIUS PRESENT IN UNSTIMULATED PAROTID SALIVA AFTER 3 DAYS MEASURED IN MG. PER 100 ML.	
Cariestat	**Zerocay**
22	30
17	18
9	27
30	42
37	35
18	37
24	31
	29
$\bar{x}_C = 22.4$	$\bar{x}_Z = 31.1$
$s_C = \sqrt{83.6} = 9.1$	$s_Z = \sqrt{51.8} = 7.2$

Our data consist of two independent samples, seven people who received Cariestat and eight people who received Zerocay, respectively. The two-sample or unpaired t-test enables us to use the information from our two samples to perform a test of our hypothesis H_O: $\mu_C = \mu_Z$. In order to do so we first calculate the sample mean and variance for each sample.

We see that

For cariestat: $\bar{x}_C = 22.4$ and $s_C^2 = 83.6$,

For zerocay: $\bar{x}_Z = 31.1$ and $s_Z^2 = 51.8$

We now consider the difference in sample means, given by:

$$\bar{x}_C - \bar{x}_Z = -8.7$$

In order to perform the t-test, we assume that the samples came from normal populations with means μ_C, μ_Z respectively and *common* unknown variance σ^2. Under these assumptions, the sample variance of the difference in sample means is given by the pooled variance $s^2_{\bar{x}_C - \bar{x}_Z}$ which is calculated using the following formula.

$$s^2_{\bar{x}_C - \bar{x}_Z} = \left(\frac{1}{n_C} + \frac{1}{n_Z}\right)\left(\frac{(n_C - 1)s_C^2 + (n_Z - 1)s_Z^2}{(n_C + n_Z - 2)}\right)$$

where n_C, n_Z are the respective sample sizes. In our example $n_C = 7$ and $n_Z = 8$. We may calculate the sample variance of the difference in sample means as

$$s^2_{\bar{x}_C - \bar{x}_Z} = \left(\frac{1}{7} + \frac{1}{8}\right)\left(\frac{6(83.6)^2 + 7(51.8)^2}{7 + 8 - 2}\right)$$

$$= (.268)\left(\frac{864.2}{13}\right) = 17.8$$

Our test statistic t is now given by the difference in sample means, divided by the standard deviation of their difference.

$$t = \frac{\bar{x}_C - \bar{x}_Z}{\sqrt{s^2 \bar{x}_C - \bar{x}_Z}} = \frac{\bar{x}_C - \bar{x}_Z}{s_{\bar{x}_C - \bar{x}_Z}}$$

Degrees of Freedom:

Under the null hypothesis our calculated t would follow a t-distribution with $(n_C + n_Z - 2)$ *degrees of freedom*. As you recall from chapter 13, degrees of freedom may be considered as the number of unconstrained units of information in the data. In this case, since we are dealing with two variances s^2_C, s^2_Z with $n_C - 1$ and $n_Z - 1$ degrees of freedom respectively, in order to calculate the pooled variance we have a total of $(n_C - 1) + (n_Z - 1) = (n_C + n_Z - 2)$ degrees of freedom.

The distribution of the calculated test statistic, if H_0 is true, follows a t-distribution, which is symmetric about zero and tends to be shaped like a normal distribution for large degrees of freedom. For small degrees of freedom, it is lower in the vicinity of the mean and has more area in the tails. As the degrees of freedom increase, the tails of the t-distribution become narrower, and its shape gets closer to that of a normal distribution with mean 0 and variance 1. The two distributions coincide when D.F. $= \infty$.

Figure 14.1

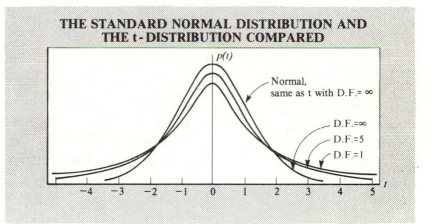

Figure 14.2

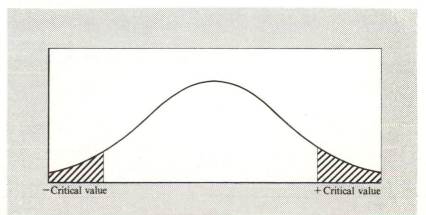

The value obtained from the t-table at a given significance level, say 5%, is called the 5% critical value. If H_O were true, the probability that two independent random samples would yield a calculated t greater than the positive critical value or less than the negative critical value, for the given degrees of freedom, would each be $2\frac{1}{2}\%$ and given by the shaded areas on either end of the graph in Figure 14.2.

Thus we see that we reject H_O if large negative or positive values are obtained for the calculated t. This is intuitively reasonable as small values of t would occur often (small differences between x_C and x_Z) if the effect of the two treatments were similar.

In the above example, our calculated t is given by

$$t = -8.7/\sqrt{17.8} = -8.7/4.22 = -2.06$$

We fix our significance level, and enter the t-table at the end of this chapter at that level of significance under the specified degrees of freedom and compare our calculated t value to the value in the table. If the absolute calculated value is greater in magnitude than the critical value, we reject our null hypothesis at the given significance level and conclude that there is a difference in the two treatments under consideration. Otherwise we do not reject H_O as there is insufficient evidence to do so, and conclude that the two treatments are equivalent.

In our example we have our calculated t equal to -2.06. If we perform the test at the 5% significance level, we see that the critical value for 13 or $(7 + 8 - 2)$ degrees of freedom is 2.16. Since the absolute value of our calculated t is less than the critical value, we do not reject the null hypothesis and conclude that there is no difference in the effect of the two vaccines on fluorocal salivarius. However, the near significance is worthy of note as it is suggestive of a difference.

Problem 1:

A study was conducted to compare the compressive strength of two types of dental amalgam alloy three minutes after trituration and condensation. Thirty-one mixes of Alloy A, a fast setting amalgam, and thirty-one mixes of Alloy B, a slower setting amalgam were tested. The results were as follows:

Table 14.2

Alloy A	Alloy B
$n_A = 31$	$n_B = 31$
$\bar{x}_A = 9,530$ psi	$\bar{x}_B = 9,420$ psi
$s_A^2 = 3,410$	$s_B^2 = 2,880$

Calculate the t-statistic and use it to determine if there is a significant difference at the .01 level between the compressive strengths of the two alloys three minutes after trituration and condensation. *(Note: Use the t-table at the end of the chapter for area in two tails. This will be explained in more detail later in the chapter.)*

Your Solution:

ONE-SAMPLE OR PAIRED T-TEST

Suppose we wanted to conduct a study to evaluate two different periodontal disease treatments. A group of ten patients is selected, each of whom has localized periodontal disease with the same severity of bone loss in both their left and right mandibular posterior sextants. One side, chosen randomly, is treated using surgical techniques, the other is given periodic dental prophylactic treatment. Two years later, the amount of apparent bone loss on the side receiving each treatment is measured and compared. The results are given in Table 14.3.

Table 14.3

CHANGES IN AMOUNT OF BONE LOSS IN MM. FROM BASELINE			
Patient Number	Surgical Treatment	Non-Surgical Treatment	Difference d_i
1	2	2	0
2	3	2	1
3	0	2	−2
4	1	1	0
5	1	0	1
6	2	3	−1
7	3	3	0
8	1	0	1
9	4	2	2
10	2	1	1
$\bar{d} = 3/10 = .3$		s.d. of $d_i = s_d = \sqrt{1.34} = 1.16$	

Here we see that the two treatments under consideration were not applied to two independent samples of patients. Instead we have one sample of 10 patients and each of the two treatments was randomly allocated to the left or right mandibular posterior sextant of each patient. This is a special situation where each treatment is applied to one of a pair of related experimental units (in this case the left and right mandibular posterior sextant of each patient). We no longer have independent samples for each treatment. We now have n matched pairs for our experimental design. In this situation we use the **one sample or paired t-test** in order to test for differences in the effects of the two treatments.

Suppose in the above example we wished to test if the average bone loss was different for the surgical and non-surgical (dental prophylactic) treatments. We consider now a single variable d_i for each patient i (i = 1, 2 . . . 10), the difference in bone loss due to the two treatments, and state our null hypothesis as H_O: $\mu_d = 0$ vs. the alternative H_1: $\mu_d \neq 0$.

We now calculate the mean $\bar{d}$ and standard deviation s_d for the given sample.

$$\bar{d} = 0.3 \text{ and } s_{\bar{d}} = 1.16$$

The t statistic for the one-sample (paired) t-test which is now based on *n-1* degrees of freedom is calculated as:

$$t = \bar{d}/s_{\bar{d}}$$

As in the unpaired t test, we enter the t-tables at a given level of significance, say 5%, for the specified degrees of freedom (n-1) and check if the calculated t exceeds the critical value obtained from the t-table in absolute magnitude. We reject H_O if it does, and conclude that the two treatments differ. If the calculated t-value is small when compared with the critical value, we do not reject H_O, and conclude that the treatments are similar. For our example the calculated t = .26. At 5% significance level, and for 9 degrees of freedom(n-1 = 9) the critical value is 2.262. Since the absolute value is smaller than the critical value, there is no evidence to contradict the null hypothesis, and we conclude that there is no difference between the effects of surgical and non-surgical treatment on bone loss.

The paired t-test is a special case of the t-test and its use should be clearly understood. The paired t-test is used *only* in situations where the experimental design clearly uses matched pairs as experimental units for the comparison of two treatments. This matching may arise in three different ways:

1) The subject serves also as the control; and measurements are taken on the variable of interest before and after treatment, or once after a placebo and once after the treatment of interest.

2) Experimental units are naturally matched, as in pairs of twins, 2 animals from the same litter, or two sides of a patient's oral cavity.

3) The experimental units are artificially matched by the clinician or researchers e.g., pairs of patients chosen and matched according to height or weight or age, etc., to ensure that treatment effects will not be confounded by any other extraneous factors.

It should be noted that the paired design is decided upon *before* any measurements have been taken, and the analysis follows the design. It may not be appropriate to pair experimental units for analysis, *after* the experiment has been conducted. By the nature of the design, we see that each treatment is repeated an equal number of times in a paired experiment. However, in a two-sample or unpaired t-test the sample sizes n_a and n_b may differ. This does *not* mean that they will always differ in size, nor that all experiments on two treatments with equal sample sizes are paired experiments! The nature of the design will clearly indicate whether the experiment was paired or unpaired.

Problem 2:

A study was done to test the difference between two drugs in lowering diastolic blood pressure. Forty subjects received Drug A and 40 subjects received Drug B. Should a paired or unpaired t-test be used to analyze the results?

Your Solution:

ONE SIDED AND TWO SIDED TESTS

We have discussed testing the hypothesis H_O: $\mu_a = \mu_b$ vs. the alternative H:$\mu_a \neq \mu_b$ for two populations with means μ_a, μ_b respectively where we have independent samples of sizes n_a, n_b respectively randomly selected from each of the two populations. We have also discussed testing H_O: $\mu_d = 0$ vs. the alternative H_1: $\mu_d \neq 0$ in the situation where we have one sample of n independent experimental pairs and each member of a pair has been subjected to one of the two treatments, and the measurements used are the differences in response for each pair. In the first case we use a **two-sample (unpaired) t-test** and in the second case a **one-sample (paired) t-test.**

We note that in both cases, the null hypothesis was two-sided in that no preference was given to the direction of the difference. Suppose now we are in a situation where we wish to test a drug C vs. a placebo, and we know from prior information that drug C is at least as good as the placebo. We are now interested in testing if drug C is *better* than the placebo. In this case, if we had two independent samples of patients on whom to test the drug we would state our null hypothesis as:

$$H_O: \mu_c \leq \mu_p \text{ vs. the alternative } H_1: \mu_c > \mu_p$$

where μ_c, μ_p are the population means for drug C and placebo respectively. Here we have a **one-sided hypothesis,** in that we indicate a direction in which we expect to see the difference. In this case, we would calculate the same statistic

$$t = \frac{\bar{x}_c - \bar{x}_p}{s_{\bar{x}_c - \bar{x}_p}}$$

but now, evidence against H_O would be given by large positive values of t (large positive values of x_c - x_p). A 5% two-sided significance level for (n_C + n_P - 2) degrees of freedom, corresponds to a 2½% one-sided significance level, since t-tables at the end of the chapter are constructed to include both tails of the t-distribution, and we are only interested in the **upper tail,** and the upper (positive) critical value. More detailed tables are published (see Documenta Geigy) which give many different percentage points. For example the two-sided 10% significance level with 13 DF is 1.771. This corresponds to a 5% one-sided test with critical value + 1.771.

Figure 14.3

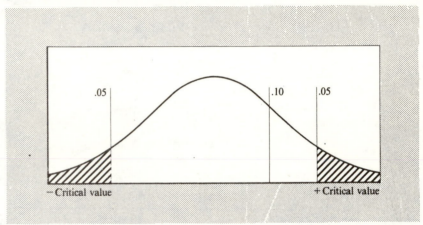

In the previous example, if we knew Zerocay was at least as good as Cariestat and we wished to test H_0: $\mu_z \le \mu c$ vs. H_1: $\mu_z > \mu_c$ at a 5%, one-sided level of significance, our critical value (for $n_c + n_z - 2 = 13$) would now be + 1.771. Since the calculated t-value was 2.06 (note that we take $\bar{x}_z - \bar{x}_c$ in the numerator and we are interested in large positive values to reject H_0: $\mu_z \le \mu_c$) we would reject the null hypothesis and conclude that Zerocay was significantly better than the placebo vaccine Cariestat.

Similarly, if we had paired data, the null hypothesis would be H_0: $\mu_d \le 0$ vs. H_1: $\mu_d > 0$ where $\mu_d = \mu_c - \mu_p$. Again for a *one-sided t-test* with n-1 degrees of freedom, at the *5% level of significance* we would refer to a two-sided t-table at the 10% level and check if the calculated t value was greater than the positive critical value. (To test at a 2½% level of significance we would refer to the table at the 5% level at the end of the chapter.)

Sometimes we may look for large **negative differences** in order to reject the null hypothesis and in this case would look to the **lower tail** of the t distribution (large negative values of the calculated t) for the one-sided test. When testing a one-sided hypothesis, the decision to use the upper or lower tail of the t distribution as the critical region (region of rejection of the null hypothesis) would depend on how the null and alternative hypothesis are stated. To use a **one-sided test at a given level of significance,** we refer to a t-table at twice that level of significance and obtain the critical value. Then we either look for values larger than the positive critical value (positive direction in alternative hypothesis) or for values smaller than the negative critical value (negative direction in alternative hypothesis) in order to reject the null hypothesis. Note that with fairly large numbers of degrees of freedom (100 or more), the t-distribution closely approximates the normal distribution. So the z tables in chapter 9 can be used to identify critical values for any significance level when the degrees of freedom are quite large (30 or more degrees of freedom may be regarded as sufficient for this approximation even though 100 DF are desirable).

CONFIDENCE INTERVALS

In chapter 10 we studied how confidence intervals could be obtained for the population mean using a normal distribution, when large samples ($n \geq 30$) were available from the population of interest. When the sample size is small ($n < 30$) we use a t distribution to obtain similar confidence intervals for the population mean.

Suppose we have a single sample of size $n < 30$ with mean $\bar{x}$ and standard error $s_{\bar{x}} = s / \sqrt{n}$. We may obtain a 95% confidence interval for the population mean μ by obtaining the 5% (100-95) critical value of a t distribution with (n-1) degrees of freedom. The 95% confidence interval for μ is now given by:

$$\bar{x} \pm t_{n-1} (5\%) \cdot s / \sqrt{n}$$

where $t_{n-1} (5\%)$ is the 5% critical value for n-1 degrees of freedom obtained from the t-table. This t value will be greater than two, the value it replaces in the normal approximation confidence interval. Hence the interval is wider than the corresponding interval using the normal distribution.

SIGNIFICANCE

Regardless of whether we are using a chi-square test, a t-test or an F-test (chapter 15), the conceptual framework for interpreting the results is the same. The calculated statistic is compared to the critical value, which is the value that cuts off the extreme 5% (or 1%) of the distribution *if* the null hypothesis is true. A mathematical determination is made as to whether any difference that has been derived is likely to be due to chance or is likely to represent a *real* difference between groups. However, statistics can never definitively prove anything and unfortunately can be manipulated easily to give misleading results. It is important when presenting data to include all the relevant information such as sample size, study design and actual p-values or appropriate test statistics so that the reader can make informed judgements as to whether or not to accept a null hypothesis.

It is also important to remember that statistical significance does not imply practical or clinical significance. When comparing two very large samples a difference between sample means of .1 missing teeth/person may be statistically significant. However, we would rarely consider this to be clinically significant. The difference between practical clinical significance and statistical significance is an important distinction, one that will often be raised by the practicing clinician.

REVIEW

1) A t-test is used for the comparison of two treatments.

2) A two-sample unpaired t-test is used when the data consists of 2 independent random samples. It assumes normal distributions and equal variances in the two underlying populations.

3) A one-sample paired t-test is used when the data consists of one random sample of paired experimental units. It assumes an underlying normal distribution.

4) Two-sided (no direction specified for a difference) and one-sided (direction specified for the difference) hypotheses may be tested using two-sided and one-sided t-tests respectively.

5) The test statistic t is calculated from the data and tested against a critical value obtained from t-tables for a given significance level α and given degrees of freedom.

6) For a two-sided test, at α significance level, refer to the table at α significance level and reject H_O if the absolute value of the calculated t is as large as the critical value in the t-table.

7) For a one-sided test of $H_O: \mu_a \leq \mu_b$ vs. $H_1: \mu_a > \mu_b$ or respectively $H_O: \mu_a > \mu_b$ vs. $H_1: \mu_a < \mu_b$) at α significance level, refer to the t-table at 2α significance level and reject H_O if the calculated t is as large as the positive critical value (or respectively as negative as the negative critical value) obtained from the t-table.

SOLUTIONS

Problem 1:

$\bar{X}_A - \bar{X}_B = 9530 - 9420 = 110$

$$s^2_{\bar{X}_A - \bar{X}_B} = (\frac{1}{n_A} + \frac{1}{n_B}) \left(\frac{(n_A-1)\, s^2_A + (n_B-1)\, s^2_B}{n_A + n_B - 2} \right)$$

$$= (\frac{1}{31} + \frac{1}{31}) (\frac{(30)(3410) + (30)(2880)}{60})$$

$$= .065\,(3145) = 204.4$$

$$t = \frac{\bar{X}_A - \bar{X}_B}{\sqrt{s^2_{\bar{X}_A - \bar{X}_B}}} = \frac{110}{\sqrt{204.4}} = 7.69$$

The critical value for t for (31 + 31 -2) = 60 = d.f. at the .01 level is 2.660. Our observed t is much larger. Therefore, we reject the null hypothesis.

Problem 2:

Not enough information has been given. If the same patients were used to test both drugs, or the patients have been matched pair-wise for age, sex, etc. by the investigator, then a paired analysis would be appropriate. If this is not the case, an unpaired analysis should be used.

POSTTEST 14

As part of a long-term study to determine the effects of aging on a healthy population, longitudinal dental data were collected on a large sample of individuals. In order to determine the comparative effects of fixed and removable prosthetic appliances on gingival health, two subsets of the larger sample were selected. One group of 16 individuals, Group A, each had a fixed 4 unit bridge spanning from tooth #28 to #31. In another group of 16 individuals, Group B, each person had a removable appliance in the same area with clasps on teeth #28 and #31. In 1970, all the individuals had a 4mm pocket depth along the mesial-buccal aspect of #31. In 1980, the pocket depth was measured in the same location. The changes from baseline were recorded as follows:

Table 14.4

Group A				Group B			
2	0	3	4	2	2	4	2
5	1	2	1	1	0	0	1
4	4	6	5	1	4	1	4
6	2	3	4	3	3	2	5

1) What is the null hypothesis in this study?
2) Using the appropriate two-sided statistical test, determine whether to reject or accept the null hypothesis at the 5% significance level.
3) Using the appropriate one-sided statistical test, determine whether to reject or accept the hypothesis that the mean change in pocket depth for Group A $\leq$ Group B at the .005 significance level. (Write down your calculations.)

5% AND 1% TWO-TAILED PERCENTAGE POINTS
OF THE T DISTRIBUTION

DF	5%	1%
1	12.7062	63.6567
2	4.3027	9.9248
3	3.1824	5.8409
4	2.7764	4.6041
5	2.5706	4.0321
6	2.4469	3.7074
7	2.3646	3.4995
8	2.3060	3.3554
9	2.2622	3.2498
10	2.2281	3.1693
11	2.2010	3.1058
12	2.1788	3.0545
13	2.1604	3.0123
14	2.1448	2.9768
15	2.1314	2.9467
16	2.1199	2.9208
17	2.1098	2.8982
18	2.1009	2.8784
19	2.0930	2.8609
20	2.0860	2.8453
21	2.0796	2.8314
22	2.0739	2.8188
23	2.0687	2.8073
24	2.0639	2.7969
25	2.0595	2.7874
26	2.0555	2.7787
27	2.0518	2.7707
28	2.0484	2.7633
29	2.0452	2.7564
30	2.0423	2.7500
40	2.0211	2.7045
50	2.0086	2.6778
60	2.0003	2.6603
70	1.9944	2.6479
80	1.9901	2.6387
90	1.9867	2.6316
100	1.9840	2.6259
Infinity	1.9600	2.5759

YOUR ANSWERS TO POSTTEST 14   Name:

CHAPTER 15

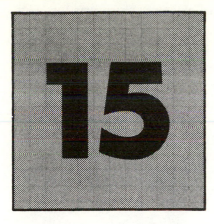

ANALYSIS OF VARIANCE AND F-TEST

INTRODUCTION

The t-test, a statistical test for the comparison of two treatment means, was described in Chapter 14. The t-test can be used, at a prescribed level of significance, to test a given hypothesis about the differences between two treatments, where the two treatment effects are measured on a continuous variable. Although comparisons of two treatments occur often, in many experimental situations we may wish to compare more than two treatments. A test for differences among three or more treatment means is provided by the **analysis of variance.** The analysis of variance and corresponding **F-test** are the analogue of the t-test for the comparison of more than two treatment means. The F-test is equivalent to the t-test when comparing two means.

OBJECTIVES

1) You will be able to formulate a hypothesis about the comparison of three or more treatment means.
2) You will be able to test this hypothesis at a given level of significance by evaluating an analysis of variance table and using an F-test.
3) In order to perform an F-test you will learn to use F tables.

HYPOTHESIS FOR THE ANALYSIS OF VARIANCE

It has been shown from various experiments that carbohydrates which are retained in the mouth for a relatively long period of time have greater cariogenic potential than those carbohydrates which are rapidly cleared from the oral cavity. A group of Swedish investigators have calculated a caries potentiality index based on the sugar concentration in saliva at different time intervals after ingesting known amounts of specific foods.

A group of dental students and their friends decided to use this methodology to determine the oral sugar clearance time of three different beverages in order to compare the cariogenic potential of these three popular thirst-quenchers. The participants were divided into three different groups, and each group would receive its specific "treatment." In this case, each group consumed a fixed quantity of either dark beer, regular beer, or a light beer which was lower in calories.

If μ_L, μ_R and μ_D are the mean oral sugar clearance times for each type of beer, light (L), regular (R) and dark (D) respectively, then we may state our null hypothesis as:

$$H_0: \mu_L = \mu_R = \mu_D$$

versus the alternative hypothesis:

H_1: the three types of beer differ from each other.

In more general terms, is there are more than 2, say K treatments, our null hypothesis becomes:

$$H_0: \mu_1 = \mu_2 = \ldots \mu_K$$

i.e. there are no differences between the treatment means.

The alternative hypothesis is that there are some differences between treatment means:

$$H_1: \text{Not all } \mu\text{'s equal.}$$

If we were comparing only two different types of beer, or any two different treatments in an experimental situation, there are two possible sources of variation. One source is due to actual differences between treatment groups, and another source is due to inherent differences encountered among individuals within each treatment group. In this experiment, the results may be due to differences in carbohydrate content of each beer, as well as differences in the salivary flow rate and saliva composition of the individual participants. In Figure 15.1, there is a large difference *between* the mean treatment effects and a small difference in the amount of variability *within* each treatment group.

Figure 15.1

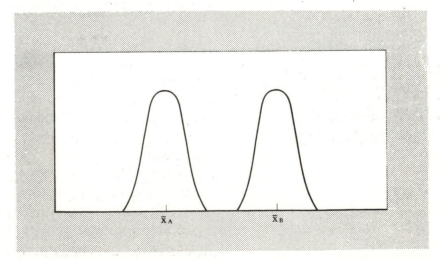

In Figure 15.2, there is the same difference *between* the mean results of two treatments but also a large amount of variance *within* each treatment group.

Figure 15.2

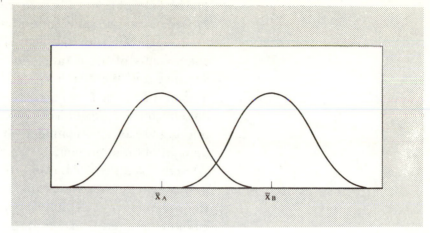

As a result, it is not as easy to draw conclusions about the difference in effects caused by the two treatments. In Figure 15.3, the situation becomes even more complicated because there are 3 different treatment groups.

Figure 15.3

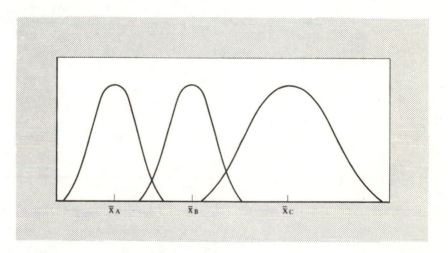

CALCULATING THE F RATIO

It is necessary to compare the **between groups** variability of the group means from a grand mean of the entire data to the total **within groups** variability called a pooled variance, of all the treatment groups. The **F ratio** does just this:

$$F = \frac{\text{Between groups variance}}{\text{Within groups variance}}$$

Getting back to our example, after the participants drink the beer and record the results, we have three independent samples available, one for each of the three treatments and we can use the information from these three samples to test our hypothesis. We could do an unpaired t test between each combination of two types of beer, but instead we would like to test all three groups at once. In order to do so, we make two assumptions. These are:

1) The data obtained for each treatment are normally distributed.

2) Data from all treatment groups have the same variance σ^2.

To proceed with the analysis, we will need to calculate the components of the F ratio. The numerator is the **between group variance** and the denominator is the **within group variance.** The numerator of the F ratio can also be interpreted to represent the amount of *biological* or *explained* variance in the data sometimes referred to as the **treatment effect** and the denominator as the amount of random chance or *unexplained* variance in the data, also referred to as the **residual effect.** The **analysis of variance** can also help to separate variation caused either by an inconsistent examiner (intra-examiner variability) or by inconsistencies among different examiners (inter-examiner variability).

Let's begin by calculating the denominator of the F ratio, the pooled within groups variance. The data for our example is as follows:

Table 15.1

GLUCOSE CONCENTRATION OF SALIVA IN mgs % AFTER ONE MINUTE

| | Treatment Group | |
L (Light Beer)	R (Regular Beer)	D (Dark Beer)
.2	.2	.2
.1	.1	.4
.1	.2	.4
.2	.3	.3
.1	.3	.4
$\bar{x}_L$ = .14	$\bar{x}_R$ = .22	$\bar{x}_D$ = .34
s^2_L = .003	s^2_R = .007	s^2_D = .008
s_L = .055	s_R = .084	s_D = .089
n_L = 5	n_R = 5	n_D = 5

For each treatment i, (i = L, R, D) we first calculate the sample mean $\bar{x}_i$ and the sample variance s_i^2 within group i. We know from previous chapters and our assumption of equal variances that each s_i^2 is an estimate of the variance σ^2. Analogous to the calculations in the two-sample t-test, presented in chapter 14, we can calculate a pooled estimate of σ^2 by pooling all the within group estimates of σ^2. Since we are now dealing with three variances, s_i^2 (i = L, R, D) each with degrees of freedom n_i-1 (i = L, R, D), to calculate the pooled within groups variance we have a total of:

$$(n_L-1) + (n_R-1) + (n_D-1) = n_L + n_R + n_D - 3 \text{ degrees of freedom}$$

By dividing the within group sum of squares (SS) by the degrees of freedom, we have an estimate of σ^2 given by the *within groups mean square (MS).*

$$MS_{within} = \frac{SS}{DF} = \frac{(n_L-1)s_L^2 + (n_R-1)s_R^2 + (n_D-1)s_D^2}{n_L + n_R + n_D - 3}$$

Substituting the appropriate values from our data set,

$$MS_{within} = \frac{(5-1)(.003) + (5-1)(.007) + (5-1)(.008)}{(5+5+5-3)}$$

$$= .072/12 = .006$$

Problem 1:

If we decided to add a fourth group to our experiment who was testing a cream ale with results of $\bar{x}_c = .27$ and $s_c = .072$ for $n = 5$, what would be the within groups mean square for all four groups?

Your Solution:

We now need to be able to calculate the numerator of the F ratio, the between groups mean square. Under the null hypothesis, the grand mean for the data from all treatment groups and all individual treatment group means are estimates of the same population mean μ. Thus, the variability of the treatment means about the grand mean provides another estimate of the common variance σ^2. The grand mean, $\overline{X}$, can be calculated as follows:

$$\overline{X} = \frac{n_L \bar{x}_L + n_R \bar{x}_R + n_D \bar{x}_D}{n_L + n_R + n_D}$$

The formula for the between groups mean square has a format similar to the within groups mean square.

$$MS_{between} = SS/DF$$

However, this SS is a bit different. It is a sum of the differences between each group mean and grand mean, squared and weighted by the number of observations in each group.

$$SS_{between} = n_L(\bar{x}_L - \overline{X})^2 + n_R(\bar{x}_R - \overline{X})^2 + n_D(\bar{x}_D - \overline{X})^2$$

For our example, the grand mean $\overline{X}$ would be equal to:

$$\frac{5(.14) + 5(.22) + 5(.34)}{(5+5+5)} = .23$$

The $SS_{between} = 5(.14-.23)^2 + 5(.22-.23)^2 + 5(.34-.23)^2 = .10$

When testing differences between groups, we are considering each treatment group as the basic unit of operation, instead of the individual data items. When we were determining the within groups variance, the degrees of freedom for each group was one less than the number of observations in that group. For the between groups variance, the number of degrees of freedom is equal to one less than the number of groups or K-1. For 3 groups there are 2 degrees of freedom.

We can now present the entire between groups mean square in a general notation.

$$MS_{between} = \sum_{i=1}^{K} \frac{n_i(\bar{x}_i - \bar{X})^2}{K-1}$$

Problem 2:

What is the value for the $MS_{between}$ for our example? What is the value of the F ratio?

Your Solution:

F-TEST

We now have two independent estimates of the same variance, σ^2. Under the null hypothesis, where there is no difference among treatments, our F-ratio will be close to unity. However, if there are real treatment differences, then the between groups variance will be greater than the within groups variance, and the resulting F-ratio will be large.

In order to test if observed treatment group differences are statistically significant we use an **F-test**. Under the null hypothesis the F ratio has an F-distribution with f_1 and f_2 degrees of freedom where

$$f_1 = K-1, \text{ and } f_2 = \sum_{i=1}^{K} n_i - K.$$

A table of the F-distribution is available at the end of this chapter for a range of values of f_1 and f_2. Critical values for different levels of significance (usually $\alpha = .05$ and $\alpha = .01$) are given in a two-way layout for values of f_1, the degrees of freedom for the between groups variance (numerator of the F-ratio), along the columns, and f_2, the degrees of freedom for the within groups variance (denominator of the F ratio) along the rows.

We first select the level of significance α, at which we wish to perform our F-test, then calculate the F ratio from our data set, and finally refer to the tabulated value at the appropriate α level for degrees of freedom f_1 and f_2. If the calculated value is greater than the tabulated value, we reject the null hypothesis at the α level of significance, since under the null hypothesis, the probability of obtaining a calculated value greater than the tabulated value is α. This entire procedure is called the one-way **analysis of variance.** Although we are interested in analyzing differences between means, we nevertheless use the **variability between means** as our measure of treatment differences - hence the name. Our calculated value is 8.33 for $f_1 = 2$ and $f_2 = 12$. At the $\alpha = .05$ level, the tabulated value is 3.89. Since our calculated value exceeds the tabulated value, we would reject our null hypothesis at this α level of significance.

Usually the results of an **analysis of variance** are summarized in an ANOVA table. An ANOVA table for our example is as follows:

Table 15.2

Source	DF	SS	MS	F	P Level
Between Groups	2	.10	.05	8.33	$p < .05$
Within Groups	12	.072	.006		
Total	14	.172			

Problem 3:
Complete the information in the following ANOVA table, for $\alpha = .05$

Table 15.3

Source	DF	SS	MS	F	P Level
Between Groups		.072			
Within Groups	18	.203			
Total	20				

Your Solution:

Let's try working through one more example before we get to the post-test:

Problem 4:
Oral hygiene index scores were recorded for three groups of non-institutionalized mentally retarded individuals. The three groups were residing in low, middle and high socioeconomic communities. Summary data are as follows:

Table 15.4

Low		Middle		High	
n_l =	21	n_m =	22	n_h =	20
$\bar{x}_l$ =	2.8	$\bar{x}_m$ =	1.6	$\bar{x}_h$ =	2.1
s_l^2 =	1.4	s_m^2 =	.4	s_h^2 =	.5

Are there significant differences among the three groups with respect to mean oral hygiene index at the p = .01 level?

Your Solution:

The analysis of variance will tell us when we can reject the null hypothesis of no differences among treatment means based on our calculated variance ratio. Unfortunately, this test will not tell us specifically which of the treatments differ. One can proceed to test for pairwise group differences using the t-test of Chapter 14 for each pairwise comparison of interest. This is acceptable if the experimenter stated which pairwise differences were of direct interest prior to searching the data. If, however, the experimenter makes multiple comparisons of pairwise treatment groups to search for differences, then some chance differences rather than real differences may arise because of performing several statistical tests. It it advisable to consult with an experienced statistician when performing multiple statistical tests.

REVIEW

1) An **F-test** is used for the comparison of three or more treatments.
2) An **analysis of variance** is a procedure by which the F-statistic or F-ratio is obtained.
3) The **F-statistic** that has been calculated is compared with a critical value F that is obtained from an F-table for a given significance level α and given degrees of freedom f_1 and f_2.
4) The null hypothesis H_0: $\mu_1 = \mu_2 \ldots = \mu_K$ is rejected at α significance level if the calculated F-statistic exceeds the critical value F.

5) The procedure for comparing k treatments ($k \geq 2$) is summarized in the analysis of variance table below:
where k = number of treatments being compared
n_i = number of observations on the ith treatment
i = 1, 2, 3, ..., k

Table 15.5

Source of Variation	Treatment Between Groups	Residual Within Groups
DF	$K - 1 = f_1$	$\sum\limits_{i=1}^{k} n_i - K = f_2$
SS	$\sum\limits_{i=1}^{k} (\bar{x}_i - \bar{X})^2\, n_i$	$\sum\limits_{i=1}^{k} (n_i - 1)\, s_i^2$
MS	$\dfrac{ss}{df} = T$	$\dfrac{ss}{df} = R$
F	$\dfrac{T}{R}$	

SOLUTIONS

Problem 1:

First you need to determine the variance since only the standard deviation was given, $s_c^2 = .005$. The new fourth term requires that n_c-1 or 4 degrees of freedom be added to the denominator and $(n_c-1)(s_c^2)$ or 4(.005) be added to the sum of squares. The new within groups mean square is $.092/16 = .006$.

Problem 2:

$MS_{between} = .10/2 = .05$.
F ratio = $MS_{between}/MS_{within} = .05/.006 = 8.33$

Problem 3:

Table 15.6

Source	DF	SS	MS	F	P Level
Between Groups	2	.072	.036	3.27	p > .05
Within Groups	18	.203	.011		
Total	20	.275			

Problem 4:

Grand mean = $\dfrac{2.8(21) + 1.6(22) + 2.1(20)}{(21 + 22 + 20)} = \dfrac{136}{63} = 2.16$

Between groups SS = $(2.8 - 2.16)^2(21) + (1.6 - 2.16)^2(22) + (2.1 - 2.16)^2(20) = 15.57$

Between groups DF = 3 - 1 = 2
Between groups MS = 15.57/2 = 7.79
Within groups SS = (20)(1.4) + (21)(.4) + 19(.5) = 45.9
Within groups DF = 21 + 22 + 20 -3 = 60
Within groups MS = 45.9/60 = .77

F ratio = 7.79/.77 = 10.12

$F_{2,60}$ = 4.98 at p = .01

Reject null hypothesis at p = .01. There is a significant difference among the three groups with respect to the mean oral hygiene index.

POSTTEST 15

A dental hygienist was evaluating the oral health status of senior citizens in three different nursing homes in his community. A periodontal index was recorded for each dentate participant. Summary statistics for each nursing home are presented below:

Table 15.7

Home A		Home B		Home C	
$\bar{x}_A$ =	1.7	$\bar{x}_B$ =	2.5	$\bar{x}_C$ =	2.3
s^2_A =	.6	s^2_B =	1.2	s^2_C =	.8
n_A =	38	n_B =	37	n_C =	48

Can you accept or reject the null hypothesis that there is no difference in mean periodontal index scores among the three nursing homes at the p = .01 level?

Please show your calculations and complete an ANOVA table. A simple yes or no answer will not be sufficient!

1% UPPER PERCENTAGE POINTS FOR THE F DISTRIBUTION

NUM DF DEN DF	1	2	3	4	5	6	7	8	9	10	20	Infinity
1	4052.18	4999.5	5403.35	5624.58	5753.65	5858.99	5928.36	5981.07	6022.47	6055.85	6208.73	6365.86
2	98.5025	99.0000	99.1662	99.2494	99.2993	99.3326	99.3564	99.3742	99.3881	99.3992	99.4492	99.4992
3	34.1162	30.8165	29.4567	28.7099	28.2371	27.9107	27.6717	27.4892	27.3452	27.2287	26.6898	26.1252
4	21.1977	18.0000	16.6944	15.9770	15.5219	15.2069	14.9758	14.7989	14.6591	14.5459	14.0196	13.4631
5	16.2582	13.2739	12.0600	11.3919	10.9670	10.6723	10.4555	10.2893	10.1578	10.0510	9.5526	9.0204
6	13.7450	10.9248	9.7795	9.1483	8.7459	8.4661	8.2600	8.1017	7.9761	7.8741	7.3958	6.8800
7	12.2464	9.5466	8.4513	7.8466	7.4604	7.1914	6.9928	6.8400	6.7188	6.6201	6.1554	5.6495
8	11.2586	8.6491	7.5910	7.0061	6.6318	6.3707	6.1776	6.0289	5.9106	5.8143	5.3591	4.8588
9	10.5614	8.0215	6.9919	6.4221	6.0569	5.8018	5.6129	5.4671	5.3511	5.2565	4.8080	4.3106
10	10.0443	7.5594	6.5523	5.9943	5.6363	5.3858	5.2001	5.0567	4.9424	4.8491	4.4054	3.9090
11	9.6461	7.2057	6.2167	5.6683	5.3160	5.0692	4.8861	4.7445	4.6315	4.5393	4.0990	3.6025
12	9.3302	6.9266	5.9525	5.4120	5.0643	4.8206	4.6395	4.4994	4.3875	4.2961	3.8584	3.3608
13	9.0738	6.7010	5.7394	5.2053	4.8616	4.6204	4.4410	4.3021	4.1911	4.1003	3.6646	3.1654
14	8.8616	6.5149	5.5639	5.0354	4.6950	4.4558	4.2779	4.1399	4.0297	3.9394	3.5052	3.0040
15	8.6831	6.3589	5.4170	4.8932	4.5556	4.3183	4.1415	4.0045	3.8948	3.8049	3.3719	2.8684
16	8.5310	6.2262	5.2922	4.7726	4.4374	4.2016	4.0259	3.8896	3.7804	3.6909	3.2587	2.7528
17	8.3998	6.1121	5.1850	4.6690	4.3359	4.1015	3.9267	3.7910	3.6822	3.5931	3.1615	2.6530
18	8.2854	6.0129	5.0919	4.5790	4.2479	4.0146	3.8406	3.7054	3.5971	3.5082	3.0771	2.5660
19	8.1850	5.9259	5.0103	4.5003	4.1708	3.9386	3.7653	3.6305	3.5225	3.4338	3.0031	2.4893
20	8.0960	5.8489	4.9382	4.4307	4.1027	3.8714	3.6987	3.5644	3.4567	3.3682	2.9377	2.4212
30	7.5625	5.3904	4.5097	4.0179	3.6990	3.4735	3.3045	3.1726	3.0665	2.9791	2.5487	2.0062
40	7.3141	5.1785	4.3126	3.8283	3.5138	3.2910	3.1238	2.9930	2.8876	2.8005	2.3689	1.8047
50	7.1706	5.0566	4.1993	3.7195	3.4077	3.1864	3.0202	2.8900	2.7850	2.6981	2.2652	1.6831
60	7.0771	4.9774	4.1259	3.6490	3.3389	3.1187	2.9531	2.8233	2.7185	2.6318	2.1978	1.6007
70	7.0114	4.9219	4.0744	3.5996	3.2907	3.0712	2.9060	2.7765	2.6719	2.5852	2.1504	1.5405
80	6.9627	4.8807	4.0363	3.5631	3.2551	3.0361	2.8713	2.7420	2.6374	2.5508	2.1153	1.4942
90	6.9251	4.8491	4.0070	3.5350	3.2276	3.0091	2.8445	2.7154	2.6109	2.5243	2.0882	1.4574
100	6.8953	4.8239	3.9837	3.5127	3.2059	2.9877	2.8233	2.6943	2.5898	2.5033	2.0666	1.4273
Infinity	6.6349	4.6052	3.7816	3.3192	3.0173	2.8020	2.6393	2.5113	2.4074	2.3209	1.8783	1.0033

5% UPPER PERCENTAGE POINTS FOR THE F DISTRIBUTION

NUM DF → DEN DF ↓	1	2	3	4	5	6	7	8	9	10	20	Infinity
1	161.448	199.5	215.707	224.583	230.162	233.986	236.768	238.883	240.543	241.882	248.013	254.314
2	18.5128	19.0000	19.1643	19.2468	19.2964	19.3295	19.3532	19.3710	19.3848	19.3959	19.4458	19.4957
3	10.1280	9.5521	9.2766	9.1172	9.0135	8.9406	8.8867	8.8452	8.8123	8.7855	8.6602	8.5265
4	7.7086	6.9443	6.5914	6.3882	6.2561	6.1631	6.0942	6.0410	5.9988	5.9644	5.8025	5.6281
5	6.6079	5.7861	5.4095	5.1922	5.0503	4.9503	4.8759	4.8183	4.7725	4.7351	4.5581	4.3650
6	5.9874	5.1433	4.7571	4.5337	4.3874	4.2839	4.2067	4.1468	4.0990	4.0600	3.8742	3.6689
7	5.5915	4.7374	4.3468	4.1203	3.9715	3.8660	3.7870	3.7257	3.6767	3.6365	3.4445	3.2298
8	5.3177	4.4590	4.0662	3.8379	3.6875	3.5806	3.5005	3.4381	3.3881	3.3472	3.1503	2.9276
9	5.1174	4.2565	3.8625	3.6331	3.4817	3.3738	3.2927	3.2296	3.1789	3.1373	2.9365	2.7067
10	4.9646	4.1028	3.7083	3.4780	3.3258	3.2172	3.1355	3.0717	3.0204	2.9782	2.7740	2.5379
11	4.8443	3.9823	3.5874	3.3567	3.2039	3.0946	3.0123	2.9480	2.8962	2.8536	2.6464	2.4045
12	4.7472	3.8853	3.4903	3.2592	3.1059	2.9961	2.9134	2.8486	2.7964	2.7534	2.5436	2.2962
13	4.6672	3.8056	3.4105	3.1791	3.0254	2.9153	2.8321	2.7669	2.7144	2.6710	2.4589	2.2064
14	4.6001	3.7389	3.3439	3.1123	2.9582	2.8477	2.7642	2.6987	2.6458	2.6022	2.3879	2.1307
15	4.5431	3.6823	3.2874	3.0556	2.9013	2.7905	2.7066	2.6408	2.5876	2.5437	2.3275	2.0659
16	4.4940	3.6337	3.2389	3.0069	2.8524	2.7413	2.6572	2.5911	2.5377	2.4935	2.2756	2.0096
17	4.4513	3.5915	3.1968	2.9647	2.8100	2.6987	2.6143	2.5480	2.4943	2.4499	2.2304	1.9604
18	4.4139	3.5546	3.1599	2.9277	2.7729	2.6613	2.5767	2.5102	2.4563	2.4117	2.1906	1.9168
19	4.3808	3.5219	3.1274	2.8951	2.7401	2.6283	2.5435	2.4768	2.4227	2.3779	2.1555	1.8780
20	4.3512	3.4928	3.0984	2.8661	2.7109	2.5990	2.5140	2.4471	2.3928	2.3479	2.1242	1.8432
30	4.1709	3.3158	2.9223	2.6896	2.5336	2.4205	2.3343	2.2662	2.2107	2.1646	1.9317	1.6223
40	4.0847	3.2317	2.8387	2.6060	2.4495	2.3359	2.2490	2.1802	2.1240	2.0772	1.8389	1.5089
50	4.0343	3.1826	2.7900	2.5572	2.4004	2.2864	2.1992	2.1299	2.0734	2.0261	1.7841	1.4383
60	4.0012	3.1504	2.7581	2.5252	2.3683	2.2541	2.1665	2.0970	2.0401	1.9926	1.7480	1.3893
70	3.9778	3.1277	2.7355	2.5027	2.3456	2.2312	2.1435	2.0737	2.0166	1.9689	1.7223	1.3529
80	3.9604	3.1108	2.7188	2.4859	2.3287	2.2142	2.1263	2.0564	1.9991	1.9512	1.7032	1.3247
90	3.9469	3.0977	2.7058	2.4729	2.3157	2.2011	2.1131	2.0430	1.9856	1.9376	1.6883	1.3020
100	3.9361	3.0873	2.6955	2.4626	2.3053	2.1906	2.1025	2.0323	1.9748	1.9267	1.6764	1.2832
Infinity	3.8415	2.9957	2.6049	2.3719	2.2141	2.0986	2.0096	1.9384	1.8799	1.8307	1.5705	1.0023

**YOUR ANSWERS
TO POSTTEST 15**

Name:

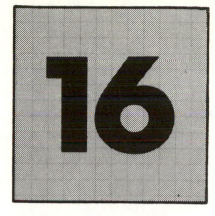

CHAPTER 16

SELECTED STATISTICAL MEASURES IN EPIDEMIOLOGY

INTRODUCTION

Epidemiology is the branch of health sciences concerned with determining the **etiology of diseases in a population by studying the distribution and determinants of disease.** Epidemiologic studies seek to identify exposure factors (genetic, environmental, or behavioral) associated with an increased (or decreased) risk of disease to help explain its observed frequency and distribution in a population and, thus provide clues to its possible etiology.

If persons with a specific factor are repeatedly identified as having an increased risk of developing a disease, then the factor is considered a risk factor of that disease. For example, in the United States more men than women contract oral cancer and, thus, male gender is a risk factor of oral cancer. Also note that maleness per se does not cause cancer; instead it increases a person's chance of developing the disease. With this clue, however, the clinician can then examine what about being male contributes to developing the disease. In this case, smoking is also a risk factor of oral cancer and it is more likely that this factor can be considered causal or contributory. Thus, a risk factor can be, but is not necessarily, a causal or contributing factor of developing the disease.

The identification of risk factors in population groups is heavily dependent upon statistics. Many general statistical methods commonly used in epidemiologic analyses are included in this book. Examples include rates such as incidence, prevalence, specificity and sensitivity; or statistical techniques such as the t-test, chi-square, correlation and regression. Some other statistical methods are more specific to epidemiology and will be the subject of this chapter. The techniques to be discussed are used either:

1) to estimate the risk of disease associated with exposure to a suspected factor or
2) to measure the potential impact of the risk factor on the population.

Whereas estimating the risk of disease provides valuable information used to help evaluate a relationship between the factor and the disease, the estimate of risk alone is not a value connoting a cause and effect association. However, if an association between a factor and disease is considered causal, measures of potential impact will reflect the expected effect of removing or changing the distribution of the exposure factor in a population. These values are important for helping to control or prevent a disease.

OBJECTIVES

1) You will be able to calculate the relative risk and the relative odds (odds ratio) and be able to distinguish between the appropriate use of each.
2) You will be able to calculate the approximate confidence interval of the odds ratio.
3) You will be able to define and calculate the population attributable risk percent.

MEASURES OF RISK

Relative Risk:

The **relative risk (RR)** is a measure of the strength of the association between an exposure to a particular factor and the risk of developing a disease. It is expressed as a ratio of the incidence rate of disease among those exposed over the incidence rate among those not exposed.

$$\text{Relative risk} = \frac{\text{Incidence rate among exposed}}{\text{Incidence rate among unexposed}}$$

The incidence rate of a disease can also be viewed as the risk of disease. Thus, the relative risk which has been defined as the ratio of two incidence rates, can also be considered to be the ratio of two risks and is also known as the **risk ratio (RR).**

$$\text{Risk ratio} = \frac{\text{Risk of disease among exposed}}{\text{Risk of disease among unexposed}}$$

The type of study which is used to assess the relationship between a disease and a suspected risk factor and yields incidence or mortality of disease is known as a **cohort** or **follow-up study.** In this type of study an appropriate population is chosen; the disease-free persons are initially classified as either exposed or not exposed. The population is then observed over a set time (usually years) and the number of cases is recorded for each exposure group. The observations from the study population may then be divided into four groups based on the presence or absence of a particular disease among those exposed and those unexposed to a suspected risk factor as follows:

Table 16.1

EXPOSURE	DISEASE		Total
	Present	Absent	
Exposed	a	b	a + b
Unexposed	c	d	c + d
Total	**a + c**	**b + d**	**N**

From Table 16.1, the incidence rate of disease among the exposed is $a/(a+b)$ and the incidence rate among the unexposed is $c/(c+d)$. Therefore, the relative risk (or risk ratio) can be computed as:

$$RR = \frac{a}{(a+b)} \Big/ \frac{c}{(c+d)} = \frac{a(c+d)}{c(a+b)}$$

If the risk ratio is equal to one, the incidence of the disease is considered unrelated to exposure status (i.e., the risk is equal for both groups). If the risk ratio is not equal to one, the factor is considered associated with the risk of disease. For instance, if the RR is found to be *greater than one,* the association is *positive;* whereas for an RR *less than one,* the association is *negative.* Remember, the RR alone is not indicative of a causal relationship between the exposure and the disease; rather it is only a measure of the risk of developing disease associated with a particular factor.

For example, in a ten-year follow-up study in the Ernakulum district of India, Gupta and coworkers (1980)[1] reported on the frequency of oral lichen planus. Initially, a representative sample of the district was examined and persons without lichen planus were classified according to their tobacco habits. The study participants were then examined annually for a ten-year period. Among males with a tobacco chewing habit the annual age-adjusted incidence was 3.7/1000 while among males without a tobacco habit the annual age-adjusted incidence was 0.6/1000. We can calculate the relative risk of developing oral lichen planus associated with exposure to tobacco chewing as follows:

$$\text{Relative risk} = \frac{\text{Incidence rate among exposed}}{\text{Incidence rate among unexposed}}$$

$$RR = \frac{3.7/1000}{0.6/1000} = 6.17$$

This means the risk of lichen planus among tobacco chewers in Ernakulum is 6.17 times the risk among those without a tobacco habit.

Odds Ratio:

Another common epidemiologic study design used to assess the relationship between a factor and a disease is the **case-control** or **case-referent study.** In this type of study, the study subjects are initially classified by disease status; the cases are those with the disease and the controls are individuals similar to the cases but without the disease. Whether a subject has been exposed to the study factor is then ascertained. Data collected from a case-control study can also be categorized into the 4 cells of the 2x2 table shown in Table 16.1 Because in a case-control study, both cases and controls represent unknown and usually different fractions of those with and without the disease in the population as a whole, $a/(a+b)$ and $c/(c+d)$ are no longer meaningful estimates of disease risk and cannot be used as such. However, when the disease is a fairly rare event in a population (as is oral cancer), $(c+d)$ is approximately equal to d and $(a+b)$ is approximately equal to b. Consequently, in a case-control study of a rare disease the relative risk becomes an estimation and is known as the *odds ratio (OR)* or *relative odds (RO)*. The formula for the odds ratio (OR) becomes:

$$\text{Estimate of relative risk} = OR = \frac{a/b}{c/d} = \frac{ad}{bc}$$

In a broader sense the odds ratio can also be interpreted as the odds of disease in exposed persons relative to the odds of disease among unexposed. The odds of exposure among the cases is a/c and the odds of exposure among the controls is b/d. The odds ratio (OR) or relative odds (RO) is:

$$OR = \frac{a/c}{b/d} = \frac{ad}{bc}$$

The risk of oral cancer associated with smoking is a good illustration of the concept of the odds. Data from a New York case-control study (Graham et al. 1977)[2] on the association of tobacco and oral cancer is presented in Table 16.2.

Table 16.2

RISK OF ORAL CANCER ASSOCIATED WITH SMOKING TOBACCO

Maximum amount of tobacco smoked/day	Oral Cancer Cases	Hospital Controls	Risk
Heavy	189	171	5.64
Light	210	243	4.41
Never	20	102	1.00
Total	**419**	**516**	

SOURCE: Graham et al. (1977)[2]

Using the formula for the odds ratio developed above, the risk of developing oral cancer in heavy smokers as compared to the risk in non-smokers may be estimated as follows:

Estimate of relative risk =

$$\frac{a(\text{exposed, disease}) \times d(\text{unexposed, no disease})}{b(\text{exposed, no disease}) \times c(\text{unexposed, disease})}$$

$$OR = \frac{189 \times 102}{171 \times 20} = 5.64$$

Therefore, these data show that for this sample, a person with oral cancer is 5.64 times more likely to be a heavy smoker than a hospital control.

Problem 1:

In a recent study by Wynder and colleagues (1983)[3], the frequency of mouthwash use was ascertained for both oral cancer patients and hospital controls. The results of the questionnaire for males only are shown in the table below.

Table 16.3

Frequency of mouthwash use	Oral Cancer Cases	Hospital Controls	Total
Daily	171	150	321
Occasional	75	94	169
Never	168	167	335
Total	**414**	**411**	**825**

SOURCE: Wynder et al. (1983)[3]

Calculate the risk of oral cancer among males associated with daily and occasional use of mouthwash.

Your Solution:

Confidence Interval for the Odds Ratio:

In chapter 10 the concept of the 95% confidence interval (CI) of $\bar{x}$ was introduced; this provides an interval which covers the true value with a 95% probability. Similarly, a confidence interval can be calculated for the odds ratio providing an interval that covers the true relative risk with 95% certainty. Thus, the 95% confidence interval can also be viewed as a two-sided test of significance at the 5% level with the following null hypothesis: the risk of disease among the exposed group is equal to the risk of disease among the nonexposed group (RR = 1).

Remember from chapter 10 that the confidence interval is based on the underlying population variance. An approximation to the variance of OR is based on transforming the OR to a natural logarithmic scale as follows:

$$\text{Natural logarithm of odds ratio} = \ln\left(\frac{ad}{bc}\right)$$

The variance of the *ln(ad/bc)* is approximated by:

$$\text{var } \ln\left(\frac{ad}{bc}\right) = \left(\frac{1}{a}\right) + \left(\frac{1}{b}\right) + \left(\frac{1}{c}\right) + \left(\frac{1}{d}\right)$$

wnere *a, b, c* and *d* represent the 4 cells presented in Table 16.1. The square root of the variance of *ln(ad/bc)* can then be used as the estimate of the standard error of *ln(ad/bc)*. By applying normal theory and transforming the limits back to the original odds ratio scale, the 95% confidence interval of the odds ratio can be represented by:

$$95\%\text{CI} = \exp\left[\ln\left(\frac{ad}{bc}\right) \pm 1.96 \sqrt{\left(\frac{1}{a}\right) + \left(\frac{1}{b}\right) + \left(\frac{1}{c}\right) + \left(\frac{1}{d}\right)}\right]$$

where $\exp = e^x = $ antilog. For example, in Table 16.2 the relative odds of developing oral cancer in heavy smokers as compared with non-smokers was estimated to be 5.64. The approximate 95% confidence interval for the odds ratio is:

$$95\%CI = \exp[\ln(5.64) \pm 1.96 \sqrt{(\tfrac{1}{189}) + (\tfrac{1}{171}) + (\tfrac{1}{20}) + (\tfrac{1}{102})}]$$

$$= \exp[1.73 \pm 0.522]$$

$$= (3.35, 9.51)$$

Thus, the 95% confidence interval for the odds ratio of 5.64 is approximately (3.35, 9.51). Because the interval does not include 1.0 (unity of the risk ratio) we can reject the null hypothesis of equal risk among the exposed and non-exposed at the five percent level of significance. It should be noted that the method described here is approximate. More accurate methods are discussed in Fleiss (1981), pp. 67-75.

Problem 2:

Using the information in Table 16.3 (Problem 1), calculate the approximate 95% confidence interval for the odds ratio associated with oral cancer and the daily use of mouthwash. Can we reject the null hypothesis of equal risk among the exposed and the nonexposed?

Your Solution:

MEASURES OF POTENTIAL IMPACT

Population Attributable Risk Percent:

The **population attributable risk percent (PAR%)** is a measure of the percent of the disease incidence in the population as a whole due to exposure to a risk factor that has been established as a disease determinant. The PAR% is also called the **etiologic fraction (EF)** and can be interpreted as the probability that any given case of the disease under study in the entire population is a result of the exposure factor. The PAR% formula used is expressed as the total incidence (I) minus the incidence of the unexposed (I_0) divided by the total incidence:

$$PAR\% = \frac{(I - I_0)}{I} \times 100\%$$

Thus, to calculate the PAR% using this formula, the incidence of the disease in the source population must be known.

Problem 3:

In a 10-year follow-up study of all residents in the Srikakulum district of India by Gupta and colleagues (1980)[1], the annual age-adjusted incidence of oral cancer among all persons was 21/100,000. Among reverse smokers the observed annual incidence was 37 cases per 100,000 as compared with a zero rate among non-smokers. Calculate the population attributable risk percent of oral cancer as a result of reverse smoking habits.

Your Solution:

REVIEW

Measures of Risk:

1) The relative risk (RR) is a measure of the strength of the association between a suspected risk factor and a disease. RR is used to help assess the relationship between a factor and a disease.

2) To determine the risk of disease in a study population, the persons are divided into four groups according to their exposure status and disease status as follows:

Table 16.4

EXPOSURE	DISEASE Present	Absent	Total
Exposed	a	b	a + b
Unexposed	c	d	c + d
Total	a + c	b + d	N

3) The RR is a ratio of the incidence of the disease in exposed persons over the incidence of the disease in unexposed persons; the relative risk is also known as the risk ratio.

4) In a cohort study, the exposure status of study subjects is known first, then the disease status is ascertained. The RR is expressed as:

$$RR = \frac{a/(a+b)}{c/(c+d)}$$

5) In a case-control study the disease status of study subjects is known first and then the exposure status is ascertained. Because the incidence of disease is not known, the RR must be estimated. The estimation of the RR is known as the relative odds (RO) or the odds ratio (OR) and is expressed as:

$$RR \approx OR = \frac{ad}{bc}$$

6) The 95% confidence interval of the odds ratio can be approximated as:

$$\exp\left[\ln\left(\frac{ad}{bc}\right) \pm 1.96 \sqrt{\left(\frac{1}{a}\right) + \left(\frac{1}{b}\right) + \left(\frac{1}{c}\right) + \left(\frac{1}{d}\right)}\right]$$

where $\exp = e^x = $ antilog.

Measures of Potential Impact:

7) Once a risk factor is established as a disease determinant, a measurement of the risk due to exposure in the entire population can be calculated to quantify the expected effect of removing the exposure factor.

8) The population attributable risk percent (PAR%) or etiologic fraction (EF) is the percent of the disease incidence in the entire population due to the exposure. The formula for estimating the EF is:

$$PAR\% = \frac{(I - I_0)}{I} \times 100\%$$

where I = incidence of disease in the entire population and I_0 = incidence of disease among the nonexposed.

SOLUTIONS

Problem 1:

This is a case-control study (persons are classified by disease status first, then exposure status is ascertained); use the odds ratio in this case. OR = ad/bc

1) Risk among never users: 1.0

2) Risk among occasional users:

$$OR = \frac{(75 \times 167)}{(94 \times 168)} = 0.79$$

3) Risk among daily users:

$$OR = \frac{(171 \times 167)}{(150 \times 168)} = 1.13$$

Problem 2:

$$OR = \frac{ad}{bc} = 1.13$$

$$95\%CI = \exp[\ln(\frac{ad}{bc}) \pm 1.96 \sqrt{(\frac{1}{a}) + (\frac{1}{b}) + (\frac{1}{c}) + (\frac{1}{d})}]$$

$$= \exp[\ln(1.13) \pm 1.96 \sqrt{(\frac{1}{171}) + (\frac{1}{150}) + (\frac{1}{168}) + (\frac{1}{167})}]$$

$$= \exp[0.122 \pm 0.307]$$

$$= (0.83, 1.54)$$

No, do not reject the null hypothesis.

Problem 3:

$$PAR\% = \frac{(I - I_0)}{I} \times 100\%$$

$$I = \text{oral cancer incidence for Srikakulum} = \frac{21}{100,000}$$

I_0 = oral cancer incidence among persons in Srikakulum without

$$\text{reverse smoking habits} = \frac{0}{100,000}$$

$$PAR\% = \frac{(21/1000,000 - 0/100,000)}{(21/100,000)} \times 100\% = 100\%$$

REFERENCES

1) Gupta, P.C., Mehta, T.S. Daftary, D.K., Pindborg, J.J. et al. Incidence rates of oral precancerous lesions in a 10-year follow-up study of Indian villages. *Community Dentistry Oral Epidemiology* 8(6):287-333, 1980.

2) Graham, S., Dayal, H., Rohrer, T., Swanson, M. et al. Dentition, diet, tobacco and alcohol in the epidemiology of oral cancer. *Journal of the National Cancer Institute* 59:1611-1618, 1977.

3) Wynder, E.L., Kabat, G., Rosenberg, S. and Levenstein, N. Oral cancer and mouthwash use. *Journal of the National Cancer Institute* 70:255-260, 1983.

4) Mashberg, A., Garfinkel, L. and Harris, S. Alcohol as a primary risk factor in oral squamous carcinoma. *CA-A Cancer Journal for Clinicians* 31:146-155, 1981.

5) Fleiss, J.L. *Statistical Methods for Rates and Proportions*. New York: John Wiley and Sons, Second Edition, 1981.

POSTTEST 16

1) In a study of oral cancer by Mashberg et al. (1981),[4] detailed drinking histories were obtained from 181 oral cancer patients and 497 hospital controls. From the results presented in Table 16.5, determine the risk associated with each level of drinking as compared with minimal drinking.

Table 16.5

Drinking Habits	Oral Cancer Cases	Hospital Controls
10 or more WEs*/day	101	133
6 – 9 WEs/day	47	52
Less than 6 WEs/day	23	106
Minimal drinking**	10	206
Total	**181**	**497**

*WEs = Whiskey equivalents = 1 oz. whiskey = 12 oz. beer ÷ 4 oz. dry wine
**Few cases were non-drinkers, therefore authors used this category as their unexposed group.
SOURCE: Mashberg et al. (1981)[4]

2) Using the data from Table 16.5, calculate the approximate 95% confidence intervals for the risk associated with drinking 10 or more whiskey equivalents a day. Using the 95% CI as a test of significance, state the null hypothesis. Can we reject the null hypothesis?

3) In a 10-year follow-up study in India, Gupta and coworkers (1980)[1] reported an annual age-adjusted incidence rate of leukoplakia (a precancerous oral lesion) among women as 1.3/100,000. The incidence among those women with a tobacco chewing habit was 3.0/1,000 whereas the incidence among those without a chewing habit equaled zero. Calculate the etiologic fraction of leukoplakia due to tobacco chewing habits, and discuss your answers.

YOUR ANSWERS TO POSTTEST 16

Name:

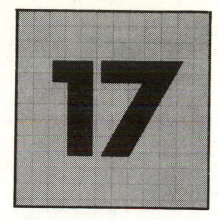

CHAPTER 17

NONPARAMETRIC STATISTICS: PAIRED AND UNPAIRED SIGNIFICANCE TESTS

INTRODUCTION

The term **parameter** refers to population measures such as μ and σ. Statistical techniques that are based on certain assumptions about the parameters of the population from which a study sample was drawn, are referred to as **parametric statistics**. For instance, the t-test and the F-test both assume that the underlying population is normally distributed with equal variances for each subpopulation. The appropriate application of parametric methods requires that these assumptions are valid.

Sometimes these distributional assumptions may be unrealistic or restrictive. If the observations are known to come from a skewed or bimodal distribution, the normality assumption is violated. Sometimes very little is known about the observations except that they are from:

1) continuous distributions, or
2) symmetric distributions, or
3) pairs of internally consistent observations, or
4) measurement scales that are ordinal or nominal rather than interval.

A group of tests which are based on minimal assumptions such as (1) through (4) above, and require little further knowledge about the observations, are known as **nonparametric** or **distribution-free** tests. These tests should be used under circumstances where the use of the equivalent parametric tests is not justified. Consequently, nonparametric tests are both useful and powerful alternatives.

Nonparametric significance tests can be grossly categorized into two groups based on whether the test and control groups are related (paired) or independent (see chapter 14). Further categorization is based on the level of measurement (nominal, ordinal, interval or ratio) used to collect the study data. Thus, the chi-square statistic is a nonparametric test for independent samples and the data can be at the nominal measurement level. *(Remember from chapter 1 that in the nominal scale the discrete categories do not need to have a quantitative relationship to each other.)* The purpose of this chapter is to introduce you to other nonparametric methods that can be used to compare paired or unpaired data at different levels of measurement.

OBJECTIVE

1) You will be able to determine when a nonparametric rather than a parametric test should be used.
2) If a nonparametric test should be used, you will be able to determine which one of the tests should be used.
3) In addition to the chi-square statistic you will be able to perform four more nonparametric significance tests.

RELATED SAMPLES

Remember from chapter 14, the test and control groups are considered paired if:

1) Each test subject also serves as a control subject, or
2) Test and controls are naturally matched as in pairs of twins or two sides of a patient's oral cavity, or
3) Each test subject has been artifically "matched" or paired on various extraneous variables with a corresponding control subject.

Significance tests which compare related groups are sometimes referred to as one-sample location tests; of the many nonparametric methods which have been developed, a few of the more common will be introduced.

McNemar's Test

McNemar's test is appropriately used to compare related samples and the data need only be at a nominal level or higher. The method can be used to evaluate the study variable (a new drug, new surgery, tobacco smoking, etc.) by comparing two matched samples. Additionally, the method can also be particularly useful for evaluating "before and after" effects and is often referred to as **McNemar's test for the significance of changes.**

To use McNemar's test for two matched samples, each subject from the test group is compared with his/her match from the control group. Because the procedure is based on the chi-square statistic, the first step is to set up a two-by-two table. The cell counts are based on the agreement or disagreement of each matched pair as follows:

Table 17.1

		Matched Control Group	
		+	−
Test Group	+	a	b
	−	c	d

where a "+" represents a subject that is "positive" with respect to the study variable (a disease, an exposure, a specific attitude, etc.) and "-" represents a subject that is "negative." To fill in the 2x2 table, each subject from the test group and the matched subject from the control group are compared for the presence (+) or absence (-) of the study variable. Each of these paired comparisons counts as one data point. If both the study subject and the control subject are positive the pair is counted in cell *a* and the comparison is considered a *tied pair*. If the test subject is positive and the control subject is negative, this *untied pair* is counted in cell *b*. Conversely, when the test subject is negative and the control subject is positive, this untied pair is counted in cell *c*. The last possibility where both the test and control subject are negative is considered tied and is counted in cell *d*.

To use McNemar's test for "before and after" effects, where the test subject is also his/her own control, the process is the same. In this case, each pair is one subject's before and after comparison and the table is constructed as follows:

Table 17.2

		After	
		+	-
Before	+	a	b
	-	c	d

Again, cells *a* and *d* represent the positive and negative tied pairs, respectively, and cells *b* and *c* represent the untied pairs.

Regardless of whether the information to fill in the 2x2 table comes from a study which used two matched groups for the comparison, or a study where the same subject acted as both the test and control, evaluation of McNemar's test is the same. For both types of studies, the null hypothesis states that for the b+c untied pairs, there are no net before-after changes; in other words, the $Pr[b] = Pr[c] = 1/2$. Thus, to calculate the test statistic for matched pairs, the cells of interest are the untied pairs only. A simple formula for assessing the null hypothesis was derived by McNemar. It is as follows:

$$\chi_1^2 = \frac{(b-c)^2}{b+c}$$

where χ_1^2 denotes a chi-square distribution with one degree of freedom. Remember, for 1 degree of freedom at the 5 percent level of significance, the null hypothesis can be rejected if the calculated chi-square value is greater than or equal to 3.84.

Example: Let's assume initially a group of 50 students were orally examined and 20 had mild gingivitis and 30 were clinically healthy. After ten weeks of intensive oral hygiene instruction, the same 50 students were examined again. Results of the second exam showed that of the original 20 with mild gingivitis only 11 could now be classified as such. In addition, among those who were initially diagnosed as clinically healthy, 5 could now be classified as having mild gingivitis. The results can be tabulated as follows:

Table 17.3

		After OH Instruction		
		(Mild gingivitis) +	(Healthy) −	Total
Before OH (Mild gingivitis) Instruction (Healthy)	+ −	11 5	9 25	20 30
Total		16	34	50

The null hypothesis states that there are no net changes in gingival health for students receiving oral hygiene instruction. To test the null hypothesis, we use McNemar's test.

$$\chi_1^2 = \frac{(b-c)^2}{b+c}$$

For observed values of b = 9 and c = 5:

$$\chi_1^2 = \frac{(9-5)^2}{9+5} = \frac{16}{14} = 1.14$$

The value of 1.14 is less than the critical value of 3.84 and so we accept the null hypothesis of no net changes.

Problem 1:

A group of 70 patients with periodontal disease were matched one to one with healthy neighborhood controls for age, sex, socioeconomic status and frequency of dental visits. The smoking habits of each matched pair were then compared. After questioning, the following results were tabulated:

Table 17.4

Periodontal Patients		Healthy Matched Controls		
		(Smokers) +	(Non-smokers) −	Total
Smokers	+	28	22	50
Non-smokers	−	2	18	20
Totals		30	40	70

State the null hypothesis and calculate the associated chi-square value for matched pairs. Can we reject the null hypothesis?

Your Solution:

Note: McNemar's test has been formulated as a two-sided test for sample sizes 10 or greater (i.e., $b+c \geqslant 10$). A one-sided p-value, p, may be more relevant for Problem 1; this would correspond to the alternative hypothesis that patients with periodontal disease were more likely to smoke than healthy matched controls. One obtains a one-sided p-value, p_1 from a two-sided p-value p_2 as follows.

1) If the difference between the two groups is in the same direction as stated in the alternative hypothesis, $p_1 = 1/2p_2$.

2) If the difference between the two groups is in the opposite direction of that stated in the null hypothesis, $p_1 = 1-1/2p_2$.

3) If the two groups are equal then $p_1 = 0.5000$. In this case $p_2 = 1.000$; note also in this case both rules 1 and 2 apply and give the same answer.

In the case of Problem 1, $p_2 < .001$ and so $p_1 < .0005$, i.e., significance, is enhanced if one adopts a one-sided strategy. For sample sizes less than 10, the exact version of the sign test for paired comparisons may be used. This is discussed in the next section. Some authors may demand $b+c \geqslant 20$ for the χ^2 version of McNemar's test to apply. However, $b+c \geqslant 10$ is adequate for most purposes.

Sign Test for Paired Comparisons

The sign test is a nonparametric method for comparing two paired samples and is appropriate for data sets where the level of measurement is at the ordinal scale or higher. *(Remember, in an ordinal scale the categories have quantitative differences and can be ranked.)* This is a very quick and easy method to carry out.

The method involves comparing each matched pair (one subject from the test group, A, with the corresponding match from the control group, B) and determining whether the direction of the difference between each pair ($A_i - B_i$) is positive (+) or negative (-). The null hypothesis states that the chance that a test group observation (A_i) is greater than a control group observation (B_i) is equal to the chance that a control group observation (B_i) is greater than a test group observation (A_i). In mathematical terms:

$$Pr[A_i > B_i] = Pr[B_i > A_i]$$

To test this hypothesis, add up the total number of times (T) observation A_i is greater than observation B_i (ignoring ties). N represents the number of paired observations that are not ties and S = N-T is the number of times observation B_i is greater than A_i. If N $\geqslant$ 10, the two-sided test statistic is analogous to that for McNemar's test. We use

$$\chi_1^2 = \frac{(T\text{-}S)^2}{T+S}$$

A one-sided test can also be carried out. The same rules discussed for McNemar's test apply when converting a two-sided p-value to a one-sided. In fact, this conversion rule is general for identifying any one-sided test when a two-sided p-value has been calculated.

Exact Sign Test with Small Sample Sizes

When N < 10 the χ^2 test statistic for the sign test loses mathematical accuracy. This is because the χ^2 distribution is really an approximation to the correct distribution. As N gets larger, the approximation gets better. When N is 100 or more the approximation is almost perfect; when N $\geqslant$ 20 the approximation is usually good; when N $\geqslant$ 10 (the rule we have used), the approximation is likely to be adequate; however, when N < 10 we cannot rely on the approximation and must use an exact expression.

Recall our notation that T is the number of times observation A_i is greater than observation B_i and S is the number of times B_i is greater than A_i. We ignore ties and so N = T + S. An exact one-sided statistical test may be constructed by using the following formula to compute P, a one-sided p-value.

(Probability of a result at least as extreme as T) =

$$P = \sum_{t=0}^{T} \binom{N}{t} \frac{1}{2^N}$$

where:

$$\binom{N}{i} = \frac{N!}{i!(N\text{-}i)!}$$

Reject the null hypothesis of equal probabilities if $P \leq 0.05$ (or any other, predetermined α).

Example: A team of dental researchers was interested in evaluating a new pain relieving medication used in endodontic therapy. The study was based on the patients' report regarding the degree of pain or discomfort during treatment using the new medication as compared with the discomfort during a separate similar occasion using the regular control medication. The degree of discomfort was based on a scale ranging from 0-3 with 0 representing no pain and 3 representing severe discomfort. There were nine patients with 2 observations each (one report about the test medication and one about the control). The results of the study are as follows:

Table 17.5

Patient ID #	Medication		Direction of Difference	Sign
	Test	Control		
1	2	0	>	+
2	3	0	>	+
3	1	1	=	0
4	3	3	=	0
5	2	0	>	+
6	0	0	=	0
7	0	1	<	−
8	3	2	>	+
9	0	1	<	−

Because the three tied pairs are ignored, $N = 6$. Four patients felt greater pain with the test medication as compared with the control medication ($T = 4$). The null hypothesis is that test and control medications are equally effective. The alternative hypothesis of interest here is that the test medication is more effective than the control. This alternative hypothesis has a direction attached to it and so requires a one-sided test. The p-value is computed by finding the probability of a result at least as extreme as the one observed, i.e., as extreme as $T = 4$. So we substitute $T = 4$ in our formula as follows:

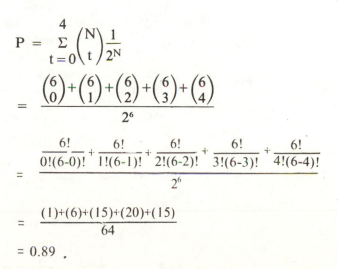

$$P = \sum_{t=0}^{4} \binom{N}{t} \frac{1}{2^N}$$

$$= \frac{\binom{6}{0} + \binom{6}{1} + \binom{6}{2} + \binom{6}{3} + \binom{6}{4}}{2^6}$$

$$= \frac{\frac{6!}{0!(6-0)!} + \frac{6!}{1!(6-1)!} + \frac{6!}{2!(6-2)!} + \frac{6!}{3!(6-3)!} + \frac{6!}{4!(6-4)!}}{2^6}$$

$$= \frac{(1)+(6)+(15)+(20)+(15)}{64}$$

$$= 0.89 .$$

The probability 0.89 is not less than 0.05, thus, do not reject the null hypothesis that the test medication and the control medication have equal probability of alleviating discomfort. Since the statistic is already a probability, it is not necessary to refer to a selected critical value in a statistical table. Note that a one-sided p-value of 0.89 implies a direction "control superior to test." One-sided p-values above 0.50 favor control and below 0.50 favor test.

Problem 2:

Cancer patients who receive head and neck radiation are very susceptible to the rapid progression of caries. A clinical trial was undertaken to evaluate the cariostatic ability of a topical application of chlorohexidine in conjunction with topical fluoride as compared with the topical application of fluoride alone. (This is a hypothetical example.) Eight patients received the combined application of chlorohexidine and fluoride on one side of the mouth and fluoride alone on the other. After two years of radiation and chemoprevention the following changes in the prevalence of caries was observed among the 8 cancer patients.

Table 17.6

Patient ID #	Change in DMFT		Direction of Sign
	Chlorohexidine & Fluoride	Fluoride only	Difference
1	0	0.9	
2	0	−0.2	
3	0.5	1.5	
4	0.2	1.3	
5	−0.3	0.4	
6	0.8	0.8	
7	0	−0.3	
8	−0.7	0.1	

Using the exact sign test, assess the null hypothesis that chlorohexidine and fluoride prevention is as effective as fluoride alone against the alternative that the combination treatment is more effectice than fluoride only.

Your Solution:

Wilcoxon Signed-Rank Test:

The **Wilcoxon signed-rank test** is another nonparametric procedure for matched pair analysis and is often considered the nonparametric equivalent of the paired t test. Like the sign test, use of the signed-rank test requires that the study variable be measured at the ordinal level or higher with the underlying assumption that the observations come from a continuous population. The Wilcoxon signed-rank test takes the sign test one step further. Not only is the direction of the differences between paired observations considered, the magnitude of those differences is now considered as well.

The first step of the procedure is to determine the differences (d_i) between each pair of observations, A_i and B_i, ignoring ties.

$$d_i = (A_i - B_i)$$

The null hypothesis states that the average difference between these paired observations is zero. To test this null hypothesis, the next step is to rank each of the differences (d_i) from low to high regardless of sign. In other words, assign the rank of 1 to the lowest absolute value of d_i, rank 2 to the next lowest absolute value, etc. If two or more values of [d_i] are the same, the rank assigned is the mid-rank value. For instance, if there are three equal observations which would all qualify as the lowest observation deserving the rank of 1, you would assign them each the mid-rank rank of $(1 + 2 + 3)/3 = 2$.

The desired two-sided test statistic, T, is equal to the smaller sum of the ranks of like-signed differences. Where T^+ equals the sum of the ranks of all positive d_i, T^- equals the sum of the ranks of all the negative d_i. T is the smaller of T^+ or T^- and is evaluated by checking the tables derived by Wilcoxon at the end of the chapter for the two-sided level of significance.

Example: Let us use the same data as in the example for the sign test (see Table 17.5). Of the nine paired observations, six did not agree. The differences between the untied pairs ($A_i - B_i = d_i$) and their corresponding ranks are:

Table 17.7

Patient ID #	d_i	Rank
1	2	4.5
2	3	6
5	2	4.5
7	−1	2
8	1	2
9	−1	2

The null hypothesis is that test and control medications are equally effective. We will use the alternative hypothesis that test and control medications are not equal (two-sided alternative).

$$N = 6 \text{ (number of untied pairs)}.$$

$$T^+ = \text{sum of the positive ranks} = 4.5 + 6 + 4.5 + 2 = 17.$$

$$T^- = \text{sum of the negative ranks} = 2 + 2 = 4.$$

$$T = \text{smaller of } T^+ \text{ and } T^- = 4.$$

If we use the Wilcoxon's table at the end of this chapter, we find that with $N = 6$ and a .05 two-sided significance level, the critical value is zero. Thus, to reject the null, our value of T must be less than or equal to this value. In this example, accept the null hypothesis. Note that we did a one-sided test when we analyzed the same data using a sign test. In the signed-rank case the corresponding one-sided test is given by using $T^+ = 17$, since the one-sided alternative hypothesis favors the test over control. If we do a one-sided signed-rank test, the critical value of zero in the Wilcoxon table corresponds to a one-sided test at the 0.025 significance level.

Problem 3:

Using the data from Table 17.6, again test the null hypothesis of equal probabilities but this time use the Wilcoxon signed-rank test.

Your Solution:

Note that the table of critical values for the Wilcoxon signed-rank test only goes up to $N = 25$ observations that are not tied. As for the sign test, there is an exact version of the signed-rank test for small sample sizes and an approximate version for large sample sizes. The approximate version is based on the normal distribution and becomes exact as sample sizes get very large. The reader is referred to Lehman[4] for more detailed discussion of the signed-rank test and the version that is appropriate for large sample sizes. At the present time you can use the sign test discussed earlier for sample sizes above 25. The only penalty is that the sign test may not be as powerful as the signed-rank test. This means that borderline significance with the sign test may achieve significance with the signed-rank test.

INDEPENDENT SAMPLES

Significance tests which compare two unmatched groups fall under the category of tests for independent samples and are also referred to as two-sample location tests. As discussed in the introduction, the chi-square test for independent samples is a nonparametric method that is used when the data are at a nominal level of measurement. In addition, for ordinal data which can be ranked there is another Wilcoxon test, namely the Wilcoxon rank-sum test. Do not confuse this with the Wilcoxon signed-rank test.

Wilcoxon Rank-Sum Test

The **Wilcoxon rank-sum test** is used to test whether two independent groups have been drawn from the same population, and is thus a useful alternative to the t-test. The Wilcoxon rank-sum is exactly equivalent to another test called the Mann-Whitney U test. The level of measurement should be ordinal or higher. The null hypothesis to be tested states that the distributions of the two independent samples are the same.

The rank-sum test first requires differentiation between the size of the two samples; n represents the number of observations in the first sample and m represents the number of observations in the second sample. All the observations from both groups (n+m observations) are ranked together from the lowest to highest. In other words, assign the value 1 to the lowest observation, the value 2 to the next lowest observation, etc. If two or more observations are the same, assign the mid-rank. Next, sum the rank values assigned to the observations in group one and label the sum R_n. Similarly, sum the ranks of the observations in the second group and label the sum R_m. The following formula can then be applied to derive a U statistic:

$$U_n = R_n - \frac{[n(n+1)]}{2}$$

$$U_m = R_m - \frac{[m(m+1)]}{2}$$

Choose U = smaller of U_n, U_m

To test the null hypothesis of equal distributions, the appropriate U is evaluated by using the tables at the end of the chapter. These tables were originally derived by Mann and Whitney. If the value of U is less than or equal to the critical value given in the table, then the null hypothesis is rejected; otherwise, it is accepted. Note that the critical values correspond to a one-sided test using $\alpha = 0.025$ or to a two-sided test using $\alpha = 0.050$. The favored treatment is most easily identified using the mean ranks R^n/n and R^m/m. Assuming the lowest rank is preferred, then the group with the lower mean rank is the favored group. Be careful to note to yourself which direction is favored as regards ranking.

Example: A periodontist was interested in testing a new promising experimental periodontal surgical treatment. Thirty patients were chosen with the same median attachment level scores who were also similar in age and socioeconomic status. The patients were randomly allocated to either the test group (received new treatment) or the control group (received standard treatment). After 12 months, the following attachment levels were recorded at reexamination:

Table 17.8

Test Group n = 12		Control Group m = 18			
Observation (mm)	Rank	Obeservation (mm)	Rank	Observation (mm)	Rank
2.9	13.5	2.7	10.5	3.1	16.0
2.8	12	3.9	29	2.6	8.5
3.2	17	3.6	23.5	2.5	6.5
2.6	8.5	2.7	10.5	3.6	23.5
2.5	6.5	2.3	3.5	2.4	5
3.8	27.5	3.4	20	3.8	27.5
4.0	30	3.0	15		
3.3	18	2.1	2		
3.4	20	2.9	13.5		
3.5	22	3.7	25.5		
2.3	3.5	3.4	20		
3.7	25.5	2.0	1		

R_n = sum of the ranks in group 1 = 204; mean rank for group 1 = 17

R_m = sum of the ranks in group 2 = 261; mean rank for group 2 = 14.5

$$U_n = 204 - [12 \times 13/2] = 126$$

$$U_m = 261 - [18 \times 19/2] = 90$$

$$U = 90$$

From the Mann-Whitney tables with sample group sizes 12 and 18, the critical value = 61. Because 90 is greater than 61, accept the null hypothesis based on a two-sided test with $\alpha = 0.050$.

Problem 4:

Suppose we hypothesized that a dental assistant's perception of the adequacy of his/her income is related to job satisfaction. A group of 23 dental assistants were queried about their income and job satisfaction. Those that viewed their income as adequate (n = 13) were placed in one group and the others (m = 10) who viewed their income as inadequate were placed in the other group. Job satisfaction was scored on a scale of 1 to 5 with 1 representing very unsatisfied and 5 as very satisfied. The following results were tabulated:

Table 17.9

	JOB SATISFACTION SCORE	
	Group 1 (Adequate Income) n = 13	Group 2 (Inadequate Income) m = 10
	5	1
	5	2
	4	3
	2	2
	4	5
	1	4
	3	1
	1	4
	2	5
	1	5
	3	
	3	
	5	

State a null hypothesis and test this hypothesis using the rank-sum test.

Your Solution:

The Mann-Whitney table enables you to compute the significance of the rank-sum statistics for sample sizes up to 20 in each group. For larger sizes, an approximate version of the test is available but not discussed here. The reader is referred to Lehman (1975) pp.5-31 for statistical details.

REVIEW

1) Whereas parametric tests are based on many underlying assumptions such as a normally distributed population and equal variances, nonparametric tests are less restrictive. Nonparametric tests are a powerful alternative to parametric tests when the data are non-normal or in studies which involve few subjects where little information is known about the population from which they were drawn.

2) Let's assume you have decided yes, nonparametrics are more appropriate for your data set. Now, which one do you choose? Learning to differentiate between them by categories can help. Nonparametric significance tests can be categorized into groups based on whether the test and control groups are paired or independent. Further categorization is based on the level of measurement. Categorization can help the researcher determine which nonparametric test is more appropriate for his/her research data.

Table 17.10

NONPARAMETRIC SIGNIFICANCE TESTS		
Level of Measurement	Related Sample One-sample location	Independent Samples Two-sample location
Nominal	McNemar's Test	X^2 Test for Independence
Ordinal	Sign Test Wilcoxon Signed-Rank	Wilcoxon Rank-Sum

3) At the nominal level, if the sample data are paired, McNemar's test is appropriate. If the samples are independent, the chi-square test is usually used.

4) At the ordinal level, we have described three tests. For paired samples the Wilcoxon signed-rank test is the nonparametric analogue of the paired t-test. However, for large data sets the sign test is quick and versatile. For independent samples, the Wilcoxon rank-sum test is usually acknowledged as a powerful nonparametric alternative to the unpaired t-test.

SOLUTIONS

Problem 1:

$$\chi_1^2 = \frac{(22-2)^2}{22+2} = \frac{400}{24} = 16.67$$

The null hypothesis states that patients with periodontal disease are as likely to smoke as other healthy matched control patients. The alternative hypothesis states that patients with periodontal disease will have a different likelihood of smoking than patients who are healthy. The calculated chi-square value is greater than the critical value of 3.84 (for 1 degree of freedom at the 5 percent level of significance). Therefore, the null hypothesis is rejected and it is concluded that periodontal patients are more likely to smoke than other matched healthy patients.

Problem 2:

Of the 8 patients, only one had a tied observation (patient #6), thus N = 7. In two cases the caries increment favored fluoride alone (patients #2 and #7), thus T = 2. Five cases favored the combination and so S = 5.

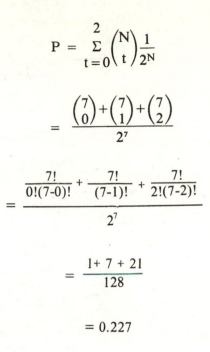

The probability of 0.227 is not less than 0.05, and so we accept the null hypothesis. Note again we have performed a one-sided test. The fact that the p-value of 0.227 is less than 0.500 implies a directional favoring of the combination.

Problem 3:

Table 17.11

Patient ID #	d_i	$|d_i|$	Rank
1	−0.9	.9	5
2	0.2	.2	1
3	−1.0	1.0	6
4	−1.1	1.1	7
5	−0.7	.7	3
6	(tied)	-	-
7	0.3	.3	2
8	−0.8	.9	4

N = 7 (number of untied pairs).

T^+ = sum of positive ranks = 1 + 2 = 3.

T^- = sum of negative ranks = 5 + 6 + 7 + 3 + 4 = 25.

T = smaller of T^+ or T^- = 3.

Using Wilcoxon's tables with N = 7 and at the 0.05 two-sided significance level, the critical value is 2. Our value of 3 is greater than 2; thus we accept the null hypothesis.

Problem 4:

The null hypothesis states that both groups of dental assistants come from the same population.

Table 17.12

	RANKS	
	Group 1	**Group 2**
	20.5	3
	20.5	7.5
	15.5	11.5
	7.5	7.5
	15.5	20.5
	3	15.5
	11.5	3
	3	15.5
	7.5	20.5
	3	20.5
	11.5	
	11.5	
	20.5	
Total	**151**	**125**

n = number of observations in group one = 13

m = number of observations in group two = 10

R_n = sum of the ranks of n = 151

R_m = sum of the ranks of m = 125

$U_n = 151 - [13(14)/2] = 60$

$U_m = 125 - [10(11)/2] = 70$

U = smaller value of U_n or U_m = 60

From the Mann-Whitney tables where n = 13 and m = 10, the critical value at the five percent significance level for two-sided test is 33. Our value of U equals 60 which is greater than 33; therefore accept the null hypothesis.

POSTTEST 17

1) An investigation was undertaken to study the possible positive association of alveolar bone loss and lifetime exposure to cigarette smoking. Radiographs were taken of 164 co-twins who were discordant on smoking habits (from each set of twins, one had high lifetime smoking exposure and the other had low exposure). The measurements for alveolar bone loss ranged from 0-4 with 0 representing no bone loss and 4 representing bone loss > 3/4 of the root length from the cementoenamel junction to the apex. State the null and alternative hypotheses for this study. Which statistical method would you use to test the null? Why?

2) Institutionalized handicapped children often have poor oral hygiene habits and are at a high risk to dental diseases. Some investigators, however, have reported a low prevalence of

gingivitis among Down's Syndrome children. A study was
conducted to compare the gingivitis experience among 8 children
with Down's Syndrome and 11 other mentally impaired children.
Gingivitis was recorded using Silness and Loe gingival index (GI)
which ranges from 0 (healthy gums) to 3 (bleeding gums). Results
of the survey were as follows:

Table 17.13

Down's Syndrome Children GI Score	Other Mentally Retarded Children GI Score
0	1
1	2
2	1
0	2
3	1
1	0
0	0
1	3
	3
	0
	2

Test the null hypothesis of no difference in the distribution of GI
scores between Down's and other mentally retarded children.

References

1) Armitage, P. *Statistical Methods in Medical Research.* New
York: John Wiley and Sons, 1971.

2) Geigy Scientific Tables, Volume 2. *Introduction to Statistics,
Statistical Tables, Mathematical Formulae.* Edited by C.
Lantner. Eighth Edition, published by Medical Education
Division, Ciba'Geigy Corporation, West Caldwell, NJ.

3) Makuc, D.M. An analysis of two complex surveys to evaluate
health status changes in North Carolina. DrPH Dissertation,
Department of Biostatistics, University of North Carolina at
Chapel Hill, 1979.

4) Lehman, E.L. *Nonparametrics: Statistical Methods Based on
Ranks.* San Francisco: Holden-Day, Inc., 123pp., 1975.

5) Fleiss, J.L. *Statistical Methods for Rates and Proportions.* New
York: John Wiley and Sons, Second Edition, 1981.

Critical Values of U in the Rank-Sum Test

For a one-tailed test $\alpha = .025$ or for a two-tailed test at $\alpha = .05$[a]

n \ m	9	10	11	12	13	14	15	16	17	18	19	20
1												
2	0	0	0	1	1	1	1	1	2	2	2	2
3	2	3	3	4	4	5	5	6	6	7	7	8
4	4	5	6	7	8	9	10	11	11	12	13	13
5	7	8	9	11	12	13	14	15	17	18	19	20
6	10	11	13	14	16	17	19	21	22	24	25	27
7	12	14	16	18	20	22	24	26	28	30	32	34
8	15	17	19	22	24	26	29	31	34	36	38	41
9	17	20	23	26	28	31	34	37	39	42	45	48
10	20	23	26	29	33	36	39	42	45	48	52	55
11	23	26	30	33	37	40	44	47	51	55	58	62
12	26	29	33	37	41	45	49	53	57	61	65	69
13	28	33	37	41	45	50	54	59	63	67	72	76
14	31	36	40	45	50	55	59	64	67	74	78	83
15	34	39	44	49	54	59	64	70	75	80	85	90
16	37	42	47	53	59	64	70	75	81	86	92	98
17	39	45	51	57	63	67	75	81	87	93	99	105
18	42	48	55	61	67	74	80	86	93	99	106	112
19	45	52	58	65	72	78	85	92	99	106	113	119
20	48	55	62	69	76	83	90	98	105	112	119	127

[a]From Tables 1, 3, 5, and 7 of Auble, D. 1953. Extended tables for the Mann-Whitney statistics. *Bulletin of the Institute of Educational Research at Indiana University*, Vol. 1, No. 2 with the permission of the publisher.

CRITICAL VALUES OF T IN THE WILCOXON (MATCHED PAIRS) SIGNED RANK TEST[a]

	Level of significance for one-tailed test		
	.025	.01	.005
N	Level of significance for two-tailed test		
	.05	.02	.01
6	0	—	—
7	2	0	—
8	4	2	0
9	6	3	2
10	8	5	3
11	11	7	5
12	14	10	7
13	17	13	10
14	21	16	13
15	25	20	16
16	30	24	20
17	35	28	23
18	40	33	28
19	46	38	32
20	52	43	38
21	59	49	43
22	66	56	49
23	73	62	55
24	81	69	61
25	89	77	68

[a]From Table 2 of Wilcoxin, F. and Wilcox, R. Revised 1964: *Some rapid approximate statistical procedures*. New York: American Cyanamid Company, p. 28. Reproduced with the permission of the American Cyanamid Company.

YOUR ANSWERS
TO POSTTEST 17

Name:

CHAPTER 18

CORRELATION AND REGRESSION

INTRODUCTION

We have so far in previous chapters considered distributions and properties of single variables. Often we are interested in the interrelationship between pairs of variables, e.g., height and weight, the level of two biochemical components in a patient's blood, periodontal disease in the left and right side of the oral cavity of a patient, etc. In these instances we are merely interested in establishing if the one variable of interest is showing a concomitant change with the other. This relationship between two variables in a population is called **correlation.** There is no assumption of a causal effect of one variable on the other. Suppose, on the other hand, we are interested in the decrease in systolic blood pressure that is attained by different doses of an antihypertensive drug. Here, changes in dose would be expected to change the decrease in blood pressure. Similarly, we may wish to see the effect of different income levels on dental care expenditures. We would assume here that a person's expenditure depended to some extent on his income. In these situations we are interested in the effect of an "independent" variable x on a "dependent" variable y. We refer to this type of relationship as **regression.** We shall discuss these two concepts of correlation and regression in this chapter.

OBJECTIVES

1) You will be able to define the **product moment correlation coefficient,** ρ, which measures the degree with which there is a linear relationship between two variables.

2) You will be able to calculate the **sample correlation coefficient, r,** which estimates ρ, from a sample of n pairs of observations.

3) You will learn about simple linear regression which models the dependency of a variable y on another variable x.

CORRELATION

In Figure 18.1a, a graph of patient income versus the ratio of the filled teeth found among the total of Decayed, Missing and Filled Teeth is presented. It is clear from this graph that income and F/DMFT ratios increase together linearly, since the scatter of points shows a marked positive linear trend. Those at higher income levels are more likely to utilize dental services and have their decayed teeth filled. Figure 18.2b shows the exact opposite relationship between income and the D/DMFT ratio: as income increases, the percent of decayed teeth decreases. It is similar to Figure 18.1a except that it has a downward slope, indicating a negative linear trend. Figure 18.1c shows a positive linear trend, but here the data are more scattered than in Figure 18.1a, showing that the linear relationship between percent of population affected by dental fluorosis and ppm fluoride is weaker than that between income and F/DMFT ratio.

Figure 18.1

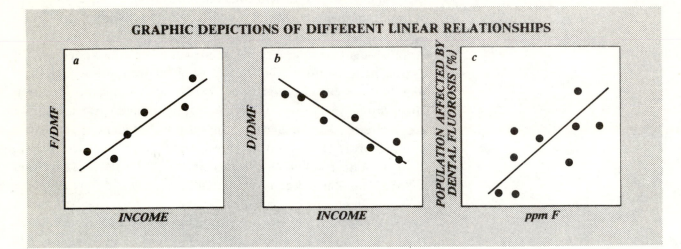

GRAPHIC DEPICTIONS OF DIFFERENT LINEAR RELATIONSHIPS

How do we quantify the magnitude of these linear relationships in order to emphasize the salient points? We define a population parameter ρ (pronounced "rho"), the **product moment correlation coefficient** between two variables x and y, having means μ_x, μ_y and standard deviations σ_x, σ_y, respectively, as

$$\rho = \sum_{i=1}^{N} \frac{(x_i-\mu_x)(y_i-\mu_y)}{N\sigma_x \sigma_y}$$

where the summation Σ denotes summation over N members of the population of (x,y)'s. ρ can take a maximum value of +1 and a minimum value of -1. Figures 18.2(a) to (e) show values of ρ for different measures of correlation between two variables.

We note that in 18.2(e), there is certainly some relationship between the two variables, but it is *not linear*. We emphasize that the product moment correlation coefficient ρ is only a measure of the degree of *linear* relationship in a two variable population, and not a measure of any other relationship.

Figure 18.2

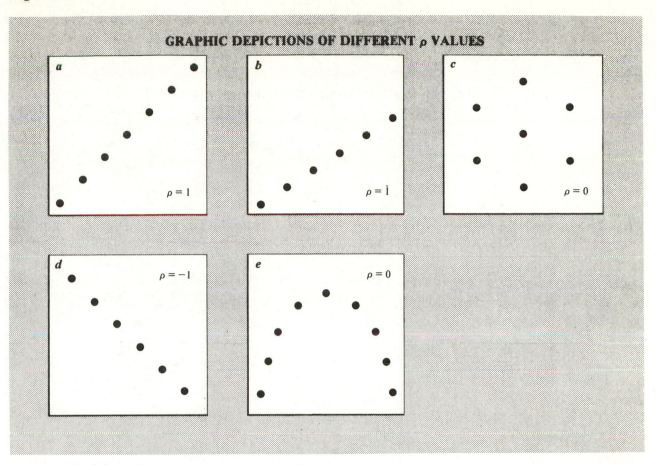

As we have discussed in chapter 10, usually we do not know population parameters, and we need to estimate them from a sample of data. Our population parameter ρ (sometimes call "Pearson's rho" after Karl Pearson) is estimated from a sample of n pairs of data, by the sample correlation coefficient r. The formula for r is given by

$$r = \frac{\Sigma(x-\bar{x})(y-\bar{y})}{\sqrt{\Sigma(x-\bar{x})^2\ \Sigma(y-\bar{y})^2}}$$

This may also be written as

$$r = \frac{\Sigma xy - n\bar{x}\bar{y}}{(n-1)s_x s_y}$$

where s_x, s_y are the sample standard deviations and $\bar{x}$, $\bar{y}$ are the sample means of the n x's and y's respectively.

Figures 18.3(a) to 18.3(f) give examples of different values of r. Note that r, like ρ, has limits +1 and -1.

If r is close to zero, it indicates that x and y bear no linear relationship to each other. There are tables available which enable one to test the hypothesis $H_0: \rho = 0$ versus the alternative $H_1: \rho \neq 0$, using the sample statistic r. Also, confidence intervals for ρ may be calculated using r, but the methods are not as straightforward as

Figure 18.3

obtaining confidence intervals for a mean. We will not discuss their construction here.

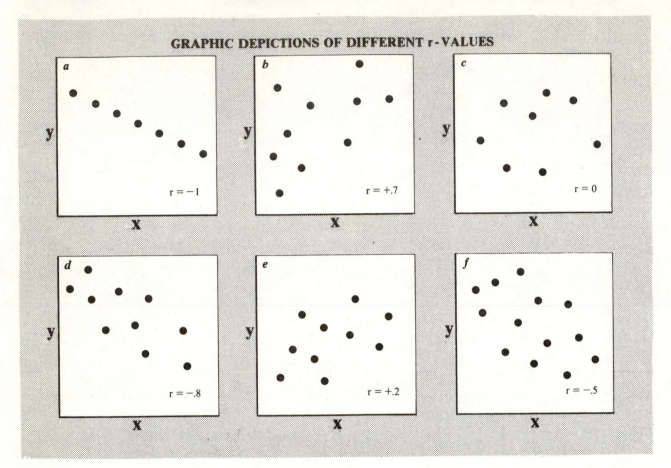

GRAPHIC DEPICTIONS OF DIFFERENT r-VALUES

Problem 1:

What is the correlation coefficient used for a population? For a sample?

Your Solution:

Problem 2:

If the relationship between two variables is indicated by $\rho = .86$, what would this indicate? What if $\rho = -.12$?

Your Solution:

Problem 3:
Determine the correlation coefficient for the two variables, x and y, where x is the dentist's gross income and y is the percentage of fixed prosthetic services among total services rendered in the practice, using the data for the six dental practices presented in Table 18.1.

Table 18.1

x (dollars)	y (percent)
70,000	.10
160,000	.60
110,000	.45
95,000	.30
150,000	.55
80,000	.15

Your Solution:

SIMPLE LINEAR REGRESSION

Suppose now, we are not interested in a correlation but in a relationship of a dependent variable y on an independent variable x. For example, we wish to measure compressive strength of fine cut amalgam at different points in time. Table 18.2 gives the compressive strength of fine cut amalgam after 5 different time intervals. The first measurement was taken after 1/2 hour and this is being considered as the baseline x = 0.

The graph of compressive strength (y) versus time (x) is presented in Figure 18.4. We see, from the graph that there definitely appears to be a linear increase in compressive strength (y) with time (x).

Table 18.2

Time Hours (x)	Comprehensive Strength psi (y)
0.0	5,310
0.5	11,210
1.0	19,470
1.5	24,190
2.0	28,320

Figure 18.4

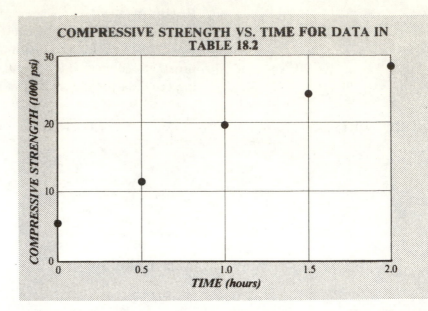

It is useful to write down a mathematical model of the functional relationship between x and y. The simplest model is a **simple linear regression model** which is expressed

$$y = \alpha + \beta x + \epsilon$$

Here, y is the observed value of the dependent variable at the value x of the independent variable. The model has two parameters; α, which is the **intercept** and β, which is the **slope,** of the line. The α and β are population parameters. The quantity, e, measures random variation due to measurement error and sampling factors which cause the observed point to be off the straight line given by $\alpha + \beta x$. The intercept α gives the value of y at x = 0 and the slope β measures the rate of change in y for unit increase in x.

How do we obtain a line which gives a good fit to a set of data? We may "eyeball" a straight line, but this is ad hoc and each person who did so would "eyeball" a slightly different line. We need to estimate our population parameters α and β as "best" as possible by using the data in our sample. One of the most common methods of estimating α and β, and thus obtaining the "best" straight line, is the **method of least squares.** In this method we calculate a and b, which estimate α and β, respectively, by obtaining a line which minimizes the sum of squared vertical deviations between the observation points and the line. We write down our predicted line as

$$\hat{y} = a + bx$$

where a and b are estimated from the data using the method of least squares and $\hat{y}$ (called "y - hat") denotes the predicted value at a given x. The differences, y-$\hat{y}$ give us the **residuals** at each point. Our goal is to minimize this difference between the observed and predicted values. We note that if our linear model fitted the data well, our residuals would be small and randomly scattered about zero. If our model was poor and our assumption of a linear relationship was wrong (either because x and y were *unrelated* or were related but *not linearly*)a graph of our residuals versus the corresponding x values would show this. The study of residuals gives helpful insight into how well we did in fitting our chosen regression model to the data.

The following equations may be employed to solve for the unknown quantities a and b. These equations are obtained using the method of least squares.

$$b = \frac{\Sigma(x-\bar{x})(y-\bar{y})}{\Sigma(x-\bar{x})^2}$$

However, since $\Sigma(x-\bar{x})(y-\bar{y}) = \Sigma xy-(\Sigma x)(\Sigma y)/n$, and $\Sigma(x-\bar{x})^2 = \Sigma x^2 - (\Sigma x)^2/n$, an easier computational form to use is:

$$b = \frac{\Sigma xy - (\Sigma x)(\Sigma y)/n}{\Sigma x^2 - (\Sigma x)^2/n} \text{ for the slope, and}$$

$$a = \bar{y} - b\bar{x} \text{ for the intercept.}$$

Table 18.3 gives the predicted $\hat{y}$'s and the residuals $(y-\hat{y})$'s for the set of data in Table 18.2. Figure 18.5 gives the regression line estimated by least squares for the same data.

Table 18.3

OBSERVED, PREDICTED AND RESIDUAL VALUES FOR THE DATA IN TABLE 18.2

Time Hours (x)	Comprehensive Strength Observed psi (y)	Predicted psi ($\hat{y}$)	Residuals (y - $\hat{y}$)
0.0	5310	5900	−590
0.5	11210	11800	−590
1.0	19470	17700	1770
1.5	24190	23600	590
2.0	28320	29500	−1180

Figure 18.5

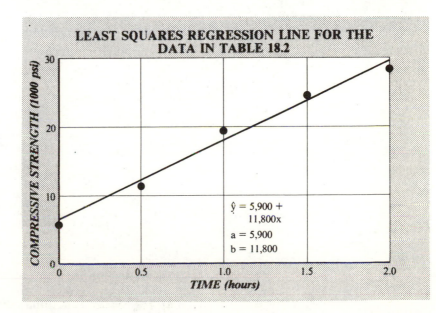

LEAST SQUARES REGRESSION LINE FOR THE DATA IN TABLE 18.2

$\hat{y} = 5,900 + 11,800x$

a = 5,900

b = 11,800

When we fit a simple linear regression we are interested in whether our x variable really does have a bearing on the behavior of y or whether it is irrelevant to y. In order to test this, we may test the hypothesis $H_0: \beta = 0$ which signifies no linear relationship, versus the alternative $H_1: \beta \neq 0$. We do this by using a t-test with n-2 DF with an estimated "b" and its estimated standard error S_b, i.e., we use $t_{n-2} = b/S_b$. The concept is similar to that discussed in chapter 14, but the statistic is slightly more complicated to compute. However, a variety of computer programs are available to do this. If the computed t is large in absolute value we reject H_0 and conclude that β is significantly different from zero and therefore that x *does* have a bearing on y.

When we consider simple linear regression, there is an underlying assumption that mean levels of y are functionally dependent on x. This dependency is not assumed in correlation. However, there is a mathematical relationship between the sample correlation coefficient r, and the estimated slope b, both of which measure a linear relationship between pairs of observations in a sample of data. This relationship is as follows.

$$b = r \cdot \frac{s_y}{s_x}$$

REVIEW

1) Correlation is a measure of the degree of linear relationship between two variables.

2) A measure of correlation between two variables x and y is given by the product moment correlation coefficient ρ of a two variable population. The population parameter ρ is estimated by the sample correlation r for a sample of size n observations (x,y).

$$r = \frac{\Sigma(x-\bar{x})(y-\bar{y})}{(n-1)\, s_x s_y} = \frac{\Sigma xy - n\bar{x}\bar{y}}{(n-1)\, s_x s_y}$$

3) r may achieve a maximum of +1 and a minimum of -1.

$$-1 \leq r \leq +1$$

4) The linear functional dependency of a variable y on another

variable x, is modeled by a simple linear regression model whose equation is:

$$y = \alpha + \beta x + \epsilon$$

where α is the intercept of the line, β is the slope and e is a measure of error or variation.

5) The method of least squares minimizes the sum of squared deviations between the observed and predicted values to estimate α and β.

6) The predicted line is given by:

$$\hat{y} = a + bx$$

where a,b estimate α, β respectively.

7) The major difference between regression and correlation is that regression implies a dependency of one variable on the other, and correlation does not.

SOLUTIONS

Problem 1:

The product moment correlation coefficient (Pearson's rho) ρ, is used for a population. The sample correlation coefficient, r, is used for a sample.

Problem 2:

The relationship between two variables x and y would be a strong, positive linear relationship if $\rho = .86$. As x increases, y would increase. If $\rho = -.12$, this would indicate a weak, negative linear relationship. As x increases, y would decrease slightly.

Problem 3:

$\bar{x} = 110,833.33$, $s_x = 36,936$, $\bar{y} = .3583$, $s_y = .21$

$\Sigma xy = 275,500$

$$r = \frac{\Sigma xy - n\bar{x}\bar{y}}{(n-1)s_x s_y}$$

$$= \frac{275,500 - (6)(110,833.33)(.3583)}{(5)(36,935)(.21)}$$

$$= \frac{37230.5}{38781.8} = .96$$

POSTTEST 18

1) During the last few years, the American Association of Dental Schools surveyed dental students to collect financial data. For the graduating classes of 1978-1982 the mean indebtedness upon graduation from dental school is presented in Table 18.4

Table 18.4

ESTIMATED INDEBTNESS OF RESPONDENTS UPON GRADUATION FROM DENTAL SCHOOL

Years of Graduation	1978	1979	1980	1981	1982
Mean indebtedness	$12,700	$15,000	$16,000	$19,700	$22,500

SOURCE: American Association of Dental Schools, *Journal of Dental Education*, Volume 44, Number 5, May, 1980, page 287.

Consider the year of graduation as the x variable and mean indebtedness as the y variable. To simplify the calculations, let 1978 = baseline 0, 1979 = 1 year, 1980 = 2 years, etc. Calculate the correlation coefficient for the relationship between these two variables.

2) In a study of the long-term effectiveness of pit and fissure sealants, selected six year old children had sealant placed on their sound, permanent first molars. These molars were examined every year for the following three years to determine whether the sealant had been completely retained, partially retained or completely lost. The percent of sealant that was completely retained at baseline and each of the following three years appears in Table 18.5.

Table 18.5

Time in Years x	Complete Retention (percent) y
0	100.0
1	76.8
2	50.0
3	32.9

Using a regression analysis, the line that best fits this data set was determined to be

$$\hat{y} = 99.1 + \left(-22.81x\right)$$

Use this equation to determine the predicted values of $\hat{y}$, and the residuals $(y-\hat{y})$ for each value of x. Plot a graph of x versus the residuals. How well does this line fit the data?

3) Now suppose another examination is conducted ten years later. At time x = 10 years, there is 3.6% complete retention. By adding this value to the regression analysis, our new "best" line becomes

$$\hat{y} = 79.73 - 8.46x$$

Use this equation to determine the predicted values of y and the residuals for each x value. How well does this line fit the data? What is a possible explanation?

YOUR ANSWERS TO POSTTEST 18

Name:

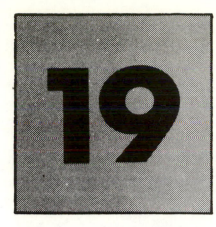

CHAPTER 19

MULTIPLE REGRESSION

INTRODUCTION

Regression may be defined as the **analysis of data to identify the main features of statistical relationships between dependent and independent variables for purposes of description, control, and prediction.** In chapter 18, which described simple linear regression, the term independent variable (denoted by x) was used. However, epidemiological and other articles may refer to independent variables using any of the following terms: predictor variable, explanatory variable, carrier or classification variable, intervening variable, control variable or effect modifier.

Multiple regression is concerned with providing a mathematical model of the linear relationship between a dependent (i.e., outcome variable) and two or more independent or predictor variables. In particular, the mean level of a dependent variable may be predicted for a set of values for the independent variables.

A multiple regression model with two independent variables may be represented as follows:

$$y = \beta_0 + \beta_1 x_1 + \beta_2 x_2 + \epsilon$$

where we use β_0 to denote the intercept term, β_1 and β_2 to denote the coefficients for the two independent variables and ϵ the sampling error.

Given that the model has some theoretical justification, the statistician attempts to estimate the β coefficients. The statistician also explores the degree to which the regression model is a good model that fits the data.

OBJECTIVES

1) You will understand the components of a multiple regression model and be able to read a table that provides these elements.
2) You will be able to code independent variables for use in a regression equation.
3) You will learn how the concepts of goodness of fit, collinearity, and outliers effect a multiple regression model.
4) You will be introduced to the process of stepwise regression in constructing a multiple regression model.

FITTING THE MULTIPLE REGRESSION EQUATION

The regression model is fitted using ordinary least squares as described in chapter 18 for simple linear regression. When several independent variables are involved, the arithmetic computations can get very lengthy, and so it is not usually practical to undertake multiple regression without the aid of a computer. Several statistical packages such as SAS, BMD, and SPSS provide comprehensive programs that perform the calculations for multiple regression. To illustrate the results that might be obtained, a regression model (see Makuc) to explain oral hygiene index (OHI) scores in terms of age, race, sex, and education is estimated as follows:

OHI-S =
$$3.23 + .008 \text{ (age)} + 0.20 \text{ (sex)} - 0.45 \text{ (race)} - 0.15 \text{ (education)}$$

Age is measured in years; sex is coded -1 = female, 1 = male; race is coded -1 = black, 1 = white; and education is measured according to number of years of school (0-20). The dependent variable, simplified oral hygiene index, is measured on a scale of 0-6, the higher score indicating more debris and calculus (See Appendix). So the model predicts a mean OHI-S of 1.72 for 30 year old male blacks with 16 years of education. This is seen as follows:

$$\text{OHI-S} = 3.23 + .008 \text{ (30)} + 0.20 \text{ (1)} - 0.45(-1) - 0.15 \text{ (16)}$$
$$= 3.23 + 0.24 + 0.2 + 0.45 - 2.4 = 1.72$$

Problem 1:
Using the model defined above, what would you predict to be the mean OHI-S score for a 50 year old white female with 14 years of education?

Your Solution:

INDICATOR VARIABLES

In the OHI-S example sex and race are variables each with two categories. They are each coded -1, 1 to indicate the categories. It is not necessary to use the codes of -1, 1; another commonly used procedure is to use the codes 0, 1.

Indicator variables coded as 0, 1 are often called dummy variables. Hence the term **dummy variable regression** is in common use. With 0, 1 dummies, the category coded zero is regarded as the reference group. It is appropriate to choose the largest or most important category (if there is one) as the reference group. If none of the categories is a compelling choice, then the reference group may be selected arbitrarily.

The question arises as to whether 0, 1 or -1, 1 indicators are preferable. In the case of categorical variables which have only two categories it is of little consequence. Sometimes it is preferable to use the reference group approach because then the coefficient for that variable can be ignored when an estimate of the dependent variable for the reference group is required. This is obvious since the coefficient must be multiplied by zero for the reference group. On the other hand, -1, 1 coding gives an average for the two groups when the corresponding term in the regression equation is ignored.

Using the codes -1, 1 an estimate of the sex effect (i.e., male-female difference) is provided by twice the coefficient for sex. This is easily seen to be correct since the difference between 1 and -1 is 2, i.e., 1-(-1) = 2. So the sex difference in the OHI-S example is estimated as 2 x 0.2 = 0.4 oral hygiene points. If the coding 0, 1 had been used, the effect of the sex variable would have been estimated directly by the sex coefficient, i.e., the regression coefficient for sex would have been 0.4 with the 0, 1 coding. It should also be noted that the estimate of the effect of the sex variable is controlled for age, race, and education effects by virtue of the multiple regression equation having four independent variables. So if 0.20 (sex) is omitted from the regression equation, the corresponding mean for 30 year old blacks with 16 years education would be estimated as 1.52. This is an average between 1.72 for males and 1.32 for females.

However, some categorical variables have more than two categories. For example, race might have been coded Black, White, Asian, Indian, Hispanic. With five categories, four indicator variables (i.e., one less than the number of categories), may be used as follows:

Table 19.1

Variable 1: Black	1 = yes	0 = no
Variable 2: White	1 = yes	0 = no
Variable 3: Asian	1 = yes	0 = no
Variable 4: Indian	1 = yes	0 = no

Note that a fifth variables for Hispanic is unnecessary, as this corresponds to variables 1-4 all being 0 = no. Moreover, Hispanic would be the reference group in this situation. To implement a multiple regression that considers five racial groups, four independent variables would have to be created in the data set and used in the regression equation. Estimates of the dependent variable for any of the race groups may be obtained by allocating appropriate values to the four variables. We have seen that Hispanic corresponds to:

Black = 0,
White = 0,
Asian = 0,
Indian = 0.

White corresponds to:

Black = 0,
White = 1,
Asian = 0,
Indian = 0.

It is recommended that 0, 1 indicator variables be used for categorical variables with more than two categories. However, one can choose between 0, 1 and -1, 1 in the dichotomous case.

Problem 2:

How would you code the following variables?

1) *Bleeding or no bleeding upon probing a specific periodontal pocket,*
2) *The seven geographic regions of the United States evaluated by the National Dental Caries Prevalence Survey 1979-1980?*

Your Solution:

STATISTICAL TESTING

The coefficients in a multiple regression model may be tested for statistical significance using F-tests. For the OHI-S example, the significance of each parameter was as follows:

Table 19.2

	$\hat{\beta}$	Standard Error	p - Value
Intercept	3.23	0.2	< .001
Age	0.008	0.003	< .004
Sex	0.20	0.03	< .001
Race	−0.45	0.06	< .001
Education	−0.15	0.01	< .001

Note that the symbol $\hat{\beta}$ (beta hat) has been used to label the estimates. Regression coefficients are usually labelled as β's by mathematicians. The hat means estimate. So beta hats are estimates of β's. Note also that standard errors for the parameters are identified; these are typically printed out in multiple regression packages. A 95% confidence interval for each regression coefficient is provided by $\beta \pm 2$ (s.e.); i.e., the estimate plus or minus two standard errors of that estimate. If the coefficient for sex is estimated as 0.20, it is likely (95% confidence) to be in the range 0.14 – 0.26. In the last column of Table 19.2, p-values for each coefficient are provided. The intercept and each of the four independent variables are highly significant. The interpretation is that each of the independent variables explains a significant portion of the variance observed in OHI-S, this significant portion is over and above that explained by the other three variables.

Problem 3:

Using the information from Table 19.3:

1) Write a multiple regression equation for the dependent variable, PI.
2) Determine the 95% confidence interval for age.
3) Indicate which independent variables are significant at the $p = .05$ level.

Table 19.3

REGRESSION ANALYSIS OF THE PERIODONTAL INDEX			
	$\hat{\beta}$	Standard Error	p – Value
Intercept	−.761	.295	.010
OHI	.188	.100	.060
Age	−.001	.004	.753
Race	.222	.065	.001
Education	.033	.018	.068
Sex	−.055	.035	.122

Your Solution:

A major problem with statistical testing that arises is whether one is allowed to test one parameter (i.e., regression coefficient) at a time or whether one must test combinations of parameters all at once. The following points are helpful in this regard.

1) Suppose one is interested in testing whether race is a significant factor in explaining variability in OHI. If race is coded as black or white, then a test of the single race coefficient is sufficient. Previously, we have seen this is significant ($p < .001$) in our example. However, if race had been coded according to the five categories, then a statistical test of any single, dummy variable for one of the race groups may not provide a sufficient statistical test

of the significance of race. It would be desirable first to test whether *all* four race parameters were jointly significant. Such a test would answer the question: Is race a significant factor explaining OHI variability? Then the separate dummy variables could be tested to see which races differ from the reference race.

Note that two seeming inconsistencies are possible:

a) Race as a whole may be significant without any individual dummy variable being significant;

b) One or more of the dummy variables may be significant without race as a whole being significant.

On further reflection, neither of these should be surprising. If race as a whole is significant, it may be that the reference group is a middle of the road group that does not differ significantly from the extremes on either side. However, the extremes differ sufficiently to make race a factor that explains OHI variability. On the other hand, if one of the extremes is the reference race, one of the other races may differ from it sufficiently to provide a significant dummy variable. However, this difference may not warrant declaring the entire racial pattern significant.

2) If one independent variable is not significant and inspection shows another independent variable is also not significant, then it may not be true that both independent variables together should be dropped from the regression equation. This is somewhat similar to 1(a) but is in the context of fitting two separate independent variables rather than categories corresponding to essentially the same variable. The section on collinearity will clarify this point further.

GOODNESS OF FIT

A common and straightforward way to assess a regression model is to calculate how well the model fits the data. Clearly, a good fitting model is likely to be more plausible than a poor fitting model. **The goodness of fit** may be measured by the **coefficient of determination.** The coefficient of determination = R^2, where R is a measure of the correlation between the dependent variable and the joint set of independent variables in the model. Regression computer programs will print out R^2 which may take on values in the range 0-1. The interpretation of R^2 is that it identifies the proportion of the variability in the dependent variable that is explained by the independent variables. So, R^2 is a proportion and takes on values in the range 0-1. If R^2 is near zero, then very little variation in the dependent variable is explained by the model. If R^2 is near unity, then the model is explaining most of the variability in the dependent variable.

There is no good rule of thumb as to how big an R^2 you should demand. In some health applications that survey humans, an R^2 of 0.2 or greater may be reasonable; i.e., you may be satisfied explaining as little 20% of the variability in the dependent variable.

In a manufacturing process, a model to predict product quality may be inadequate unless R^2 is 0.7 or more. It is best to interpret a *good* or *bad* R^2 according to previous work of a similar nature. However, it is important that the joint set of independent variables in the model explain a statistically significant proportion of the variance of the dependent variable, i.e., it is important that R^2 be significantly different from zero. Such a test of the regression model is usually provided as output from a regression computer package.

COLLINEARITY

When two or more independent variables are mutually and highly correlated, the predictive power of one of the independent variables is only partially distinguishable from the predictive power of the correlated variable (or group of variables). In this situation, the statistical technique of least squares has difficulty deciding how much predictive ability to allocate to one or other of the independent variables. Such a **collinear** situation complicates interpretation because the analyst is often interested in the incremental influence of a particular independent variable when the other factors are controlled. If the other factors have a tendency to be collinear with the independent variable of interest, then the notion of incremental influence becomes a difficult one to decide because it is dependent on the multiple regression model used.

For example, the OHI regression model referred to previously has age, sex, race, and education as independent variables. If income was included as a fifth variable, it would likely be collinear with education. In other words, the correlation between education and income would complicate the interpretation regarding the marginal effect of education. This marginal effect might be very low if income was in the model because once income is controlled for, the additional explaining power of education may be small. This creates something of a problem as regards defining what we mean by the marginal effect of education. As we have seen, this marginal effect is large with respect to the regression model with four independent variables.

In general, a reasonable approach to this problem is to avoid putting collinear variables in a regression model; i.e., in our example use income or eduation but not both. Another approach might be to construct an index that measured the joint effects of income and education (e.g., income + education using appropriate units) and use the index in the regression model. As a rule of thumb, variables that are pairwise correlated with $R > 0.7$ should not both be included in a regression model.

Problem 4:
Explain what is meant by collinearity.

Your Solution:

INFLUENTIAL DATA POINTS

Some data points influence the estimates of the regression coefficients far more than others. It is important to recognize this as it may be inappropriate for a regression coefficient to be dominated by just one or two elements in the sample. Points close to mean values are of least influence on the regression coefficients. Points extreme from mean values have the most influence on the regression coefficients. So statistical outliers are good candidates for careful review to see if they are unduly influencing the regression coefficients. An outlier may be any point beyond 3 standard deviations from the mean.

If an outlier is detected that appears to be influential, an appropriate strategy would be to fit the regression model a second time eliminating the suspicious point. Review of the *change* in one or more of the regression coefficients will identify the influence of this one point. The next step is to decide what to do with the influential point. It cannot just be eliminated because the point may be valid and exerting appropriate influence. The safest tactic is to make sure that the values associated with the item are correct and also confirm that it can be regarded as part of a reasonably homogeneous sample. If there is considerable doubt about either of these issues, the data point should probably be eliminated. Otherwise, the safest ploy would be to include the point but comment on the degree of influence the single value exerted. Similar remarks apply if two or more points are jointly influential.

Problem 5:

Where are data points that have the most and least influence on regression coefficients most likely to be located?

Your Solution:

ERROR OF MEASUREMENT IN INDEPENDENT VARIABLES

Multiple regression assumes that the dependent variable may be measured with error but does not assume that errors of measurement are present for any of the independent variables. If the latter is the case, biased estimates of regression coefficients can result. It would be prudent to consult with an experienced statistician if this "error in variables" problem arises.

STEPWISE REGRESSION

One is often faced with the situation of having many independent variables and wishing to explore which set of variables best explain variability in the dependent variable. **Stepwise regression** is well suited to this task. The idea is to choose the first independent variable on the basis of which one explains the most variation in the dependent variable. Then a second variable is added according to next most variance explained. The procedure continues in a stepwise fashion; hence the name.

The forward selection procedure can be amplified by backward elimination. It may be that one of the variables ceases to be a good explainer of variability when other related variables ascend to the model. The OHI example may provide an illustration. If a stepwise analysis had been performed, income may enter at the fifth step. However, education may cease to be an important explainer of extra variance once age, sex, race, and income are in the model. Backward elimination of unnecessary variables can be included in a stepwise procedure in order to achieve a parsimonious model. More detailed descriptions of stepwise algorithms should be available in the computer package that you use.

Probably the most important assumption of a multiple regression equation is that the model itself has some theoretical justification. It is not wise to rely solely on statistical computations to generate a model. Instead, there is need for a careful interplay between the substantive knowledge in the area of application and the facts being communicated by the data set at hand.

REVIEW

1) Multiple regression provides a mathematical model of the linear relationship between a dependent (outcome) variable and two or more independent or predictor variables.
2) Model with two independent variables:

$$y = \beta_0 + \beta_1 \chi_1 + \beta_2 \chi_2 + e$$

The regression coefficients may be tested for statistical significance using F-tests.
3) Dummy variable regression uses indicator variables coded as 0, 1 to distinguish many categories where 0 can be regarded as the reference group. Dichotomous variables can be coded -1, 1.

4) The goodness of fit of a model may be measured by the coefficient of determination, R^2. In a good fitting model, there is close agreement between expected and observed values and R^2 approaches 1.

5) When two or more independent variables are highly correlated, the predictive power of one of the independent variables is only partially distinguishable from the predictive power of the correlated variable (or groups of variables). Such variables are said to be **collinear**.

6) In **stepwise regression**, the independent variables are chosen on the basis of the amount of variation they explain in the dependent variable. In **forward selection**, the variable which explains the most is chosen first, the greatest amount over and above that explained by the first is chosen second, and so forth. However, the regression coefficients change depending on what else is in the model so that the addition of a new variable may cause a previously added variable to lose significance. In **backward selection**, the model begins with all the independent variables. The variables are deleted one at a time to see if they significantly reduce the fit of the model. Stepwise selection includes both forward and backward selection to obtain the model that best balances parsimony and goodness of fit.

SOLUTIONS

Problem 1:

OHI = 3.23 + .008(50) + .20(-1) - 0.45(1) - 0.15(14)
= 3.23 + .40 - .20 - 0.45 - 2.1 = .88

Problem 2:

1) Either 0, 1 or -1, 1 can be used to code presence or absence of bleeding upon probing, depending on how the information will be used.

2) Six variables are needed to describe seven geographic regions:
Variable 1, Region 1, 1 = yes, 0 = no
Variable 2, Region 2, 1 = yes, 0 = no
Variable 3, Region 3, 1 = yes, 0 = no
Variable 4, Region 4, 1 = yes, 0 = no
Variable 5, Region 5, 1 = yes, 0 = no
Varaible 6, Region 6, 1 = yes, 0 = no
Region 7, Variables all coded 0.

Problem 3:

1) PI = -.761 + .188 (OHI) - .001 (Age) + .222 (Race) + .033 (Education) - .055 (Sex)

2) 95% CI (age) = -.001 $\pm$ 2(.004) = -.009 to .007

3) Race is significant at the p = .05 level.

Problem 4:

When two or more independent variables are highly correlated with each other and with the dependent variable, it is difficult to determine which of the independent variables should be considered as having the better predictive power.

Problem 5:

Data points that are outliers more than 3 standard deviations from the mean exert the most influence on regression coefficients and data points that are close to or at the mean, the least influence.

POSTTEST 19

Select the correct answers:

1) Multiple regression can be used
    a) to explain the effects of many independent variables on a particular outcome variable.
    b) to determine which of many variables have the most influence on a particular outcome variable.
    c) to predict the value of the mean level of a dependent variable given possible values of independent variables.
    d) all of the above.

2) To develop the best regression model, which of the following statements are true?
    a) A large Coefficient of Determination is desirable.
    b) Additional variables should significantly improve the goodness of fit.
    c) Outliers should always be eliminated.
    d) In general, collinear variables should be included.
    e) Use forward and not backward selection.

YOUR ANSWERS
TO POSTTEST 19

Name:

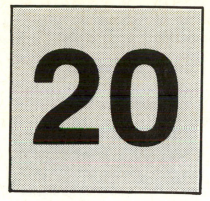

CHAPTER 20

THE RESEARCH PROTOCOL

INTRODUCTION

Now that you have completed all of the chapters on data analysis, you should be curious, or perhaps even frustrated, because you do not quite see how data analysis fits into the whole research project. In this chapter we will go through the steps in writing a research protocol and conducting a research project. First, the uses of a research protocol will be reviewed. Then, each of the major sections of a research protocol will be described using dental research examples.

OBJECTIVES

1) You will know at least four reasons for writing a research protocol.
2) You will be able to list the seven primary sections of a research protocol and know the sequence of steps in a research project.
3) You will be able to write an outline of a research protocol for a dental research project.
4) You will be able to evaluate a research protocol and a journal article.

USES OF A PROTOCOL

When you know the uses of a research protocol you will understand the logical sequence of the major sections of a research protocol. We will first identify these uses — or reasons for writing a research protocol — and then see how they are linked to the different sections within the protocol itself.

There are four main uses of a research protocol. Knowing these uses will help you clarify the project and improve your ability to communicate it to others (such as other researchers and funding agencies). A research protocol is used to tell others:

1) why the research is needed;
2) what procedures must be conducted;
3) how procedures will be carried out; and
4) what results you expect from the analysis.

For a shorthand method of committing the *uses of a protocol* to memory, the following key words may help:

Why,
What,
How, and
So what?

An aside: If you are familiar with writing skills or have ever taken a communications course, you probably recognize these key words. It is not a coincidence that these reasons for writing a research protocol are similar to concepts which are considered to be communication skills or characteristics of a journal article, or in other disciplines, the fundamentals of program planning and management. Writing and communication skills are generally the same regardless of the subject matter.

The four main uses for a research protocol can be turned around and applied by you in evaluating any research journal article. When reading an article, ask yourself the following four questions:

1) *Why is this article important?* Are the research question and study results important?

2) *What do the authors say?* What are the research question and study results?

3) *How do they know?* Is the research design appropriate and are the data collection methods valid?

4) *So what?* Is there any significance to the findings, or do the results really add to existing knowledge?

Now, before you think this is too easy, let's go over the uses of a research protocol one more time.

Problem 1:
Without looking back to find the answer, list the four main uses of a research protocol.

Your Solution:

Now go on to the next section to see how the major sections of a research protocol match up with these uses.

SECTIONS IN THE PROTOCOL

A research protocol has *seven* major sections which, if followed, tell the why, what, how, and so what of the project. The finished protocol will serve to explain the purpose for asking the research questions and provide an explicit plan for conducting the research project. This plan will identify the resources needed to carry out the research and should be in sufficient detail so that the same project can be conducted again by another investigator in another time and place. The seven sections are as follows.

1. *Background and Problem*

The most common mistake committed by many new investigators is the omission of this first critical step. The worse example of such early trouble is: "I didn't do a review of the literature because I haven't decided on my specific research question yet."

WRONG!*#@*!#

First, a general problem is realized. It could be a basic science (biochemical, bacteriological, genetic, etc.), clinical (diagnostic test, treatment efficacy, patient management), or health care delivery system (health care financing or organization of services) problem. Next, a search is made of all the literature that bears upon the general problem. It is from this critical review of the literature that the final specific research question is generated. Thus, the specific research question to be studied in your research project is a **result** of the review of the literature, not vice versa. It is the investigator's responsibility to know the relevant work of other researchers that is related to the specific research question under study. This section includes:

— a statement of the general problem that has stimulated the inquiry;

— the reasons for undertaking and significance of the research (a convincing argument that catches the reader's scientific interest);

— a critical review of the relevant literature; and

— a list of references that documents the review.

It is important to understand that the review of the literature should really be a critical review. This means that the design, measures, data collection, and analysis of each of the relevant previous studies must be evaluated for validity and reliability. Your specific research question is only required to be responsive to the previous studies that are found to have been valid designs, procedures and analyses.

2. *Objectives or Hypotheses*

This section is short, but indispensable. Hypotheses should be written if at all possible. Too often a research project is initiated without first articulating the expected results. You should have some idea about the outcome. These expectations are then reflected in the hypotheses. Studies that test cause and effect relationships of specified substances or phenomena are required to state a hypothesis regarding expected relationships. If the research is exploratory or descriptive, a hypothesis may be inappropriate because not enough is known about the variables under study. Objectives should be written for these studies.

The Null Hypothesis: A statistical framework for stating a hypothesis is in the form of a null hypothesis. Formulating a null hypothesis is discussed in Chapter 11. Investigators sometimes prefer to state the hypotheses in a positive manner, identifying expectations of the results. This method is acceptable, but remember that statistical tests are formulated in an attempt to reject the underlying null hypothesis.

3. *Research Design*

Specification of the research objectives leads to the necessity of defining the population under study. Population here does not necessarily refer to people; it means the kinds of units or elements from which the data are to be obtained. It could be test tubes, or slides for microscopic examination, or people. If the research requires a sample from this population, see Chapter 8 for the methods to be employed. If the research is intended to test the cause and effect relationship between various phenomena, then some kind of experimental or quasi-experimental design would be appropriate. The next chapter on clinical trials covers the three major classes of experimental designs.

There are two primary classes of research designs that are used in the overwhelming majority of research in the health sciences. One is *survey research,* which is often applied in the form of epidemiologic research in its medical context, and includes research projects that are designed to describe the distribution of a specified factor within a specified population. The second is *experimental research* which is used to test cause and effect relationships. Experimental research designs are almost the *sine qua non* of biomedical research. The scientific questions are quite specific and the overwhelming majority of biomedical research projects attempt to discover the effect of one element, substance or phenomenon upon another element, substance or phenomenon. The most frequently used experimental research designs are described in Chapter 21.

After the design is clearly described, procedures should also be written out for:
— pretesting the data collection methods;
— training the persons who will collect the data; and
— describing the physical procedures (who, when, where) for collecting the data when the study period begins.

4. *Data to be Collected*

Knowing the specific research design and being able to state the objectives or hypotheses sets the stage for deciding upon the data that need to be collected. A good first step is to make a list of each variable and measurement for which data are required. This list should include all of the data that will be required to test the stated hypotheses or accomplish the study objectives. The naming of each variable is called the *conceptual definition;* describing precisely how each variable is going to be measured is called the *operational definition.*

The data collection section should clearly describe how each item of data will be obtained, including a specification of who is responsible for obtaining, recording and storing each data item. This section can include a copy of the forms to be used for data collection, or the initial draft of such a form.

5. *Data Analysis and Reporting Plans*

The research protocol should include a detailed description of the data management, analysis and reporting procedures. A short check list of the content of this section includes how the data will be:

a) checked for accuracy and completeness;
b) summarized by descriptive statistics;
c) analyzed with tests of significance; and
d) presented in tables, figures and graphs.

It is not necessary for the protocol to contain a lengthy description of these procedures, but it is advisable that the investigators demonstrate their knowledge of these important steps by mentioning them within the data management and analysis section of the protocol.

A critical step that is sometimes underestimated in its time requirements occurs at this point in the research project. It is the *interpretation* of results, *secondary analysis* and subsequent *report writing.* The amount of time needed to think about the results and understand them in view of previous studies is often far greater than the new investigator expects or plans. In fact, it may well be that the time required for interpretation and report writing is so much greater than anticipated that the pressure to move on to the next project, patient, or administrative task preempts the publication of a well-written final report. This state of affairs is regrettable and should be recognized by researchers and funding institutions at the time of writing the research protocol.

Outline of final report: The basic outline of a written report includes the five sections just presented plus the *results, discussion* and *summary,* and *conclusions.* A typical report will have the following outline.

1) *Introduction* – to summarize the objectives, previous studies, and relevant clinical background of the trial.
2) *Methods* – to describe the experimental *design* and conduct of the trial, including the measurement methods and the *data collection* procedures; and to summarize the statistical methods used in the *analysis* of results (complete references should be provided).
3) *Results* – to include a complete set of tables and figures describing patients who participated in the study and summarizing all findings related to efficacy, safety and other research questions. These data should be presented in a clear, descriptive manner with a concise narrative to highlight important findings.
4) *Discussion* – to provide a careful interpretation of the meaning of descriptive and inferential results relative to the pre-defined objectives of the study. Comparisons with previous studies are made, threats to validity and reliability are discussed, and alternative explanations of the findings are considered.
5) *Summary and Conclusions* – to provide an overview of the entire study. The conclusions should answer the basic question raised in the objectives. Is the new preventive, diagnostic method or treatments regimen safe and effective as compared to the standard procedure?

6. *Work Schedule*

The first five sections of the protocol represent the scientific planning for the research project. The sixth and seventh sections represent the administrative planning for the project. The entire schedule is often laid out in a single table in which the activities within the principal phases of the project are listed down the left hand column and the months in which each activity will take place are listed across the top row. There is little guesswork in deciding what activities should be listed in the column. Just read back over your research protocol and include each of the stated or implied activities within the first six sections. Each activity should have a starting and stopping date. Constructing the work schedule will force you to realize that while certain activities can be carried out simultaneously, some sets of activities are contingent on others being accomplished first. Thus, planning the schedule will enable you to plan how long the project will take with all of these constraints, and within your particular organization. You may need to include some project management activities such as planning time and the administration time that is required to conduct the project within your institution. For example, personnel appointments and financial accounting procedures are usually required by the education institution, corporation, or government agency for which you are working.

A mini version of a typical work schedule might look something like the one below. This type of work schedule is often called a Gant Chart after the person from whom the idea originated. Each of the nine work activities listed can be broken down into tasks. For example, the activity of hiring personnel would include tasks such as writing job descriptions, advertising positions, and interviewing candidates.

Annual Calendar

Work Activities	Jan.	Feb.	Mar.	Apr.	May	June	July	Aug.	Sep.	Oct.	Nov.	Dec.
Hire personnel	●━━━━━━●											
Pretest methods		●━━●										
Print forms			●━━●									
Data collection				●━━━━━━●								
Data entry					●━━━━━━●							
Data analysis						●━━●		●━●		●━●		
Interpretation							●━●		●━●		●━●	
Report writing						●━━●				●━━━━━━━━━●		
Financial audits			●━●			●━●			●━●			●━●

7. *Budget and Budget Justification*

The section of the protocol that demonstrates your understanding of the effort necessary for completing the project is your description of resources needed. This section can usually be completely contained in the budget and budget justification which explains how each cost item presented in the budget has been derived.

Page 250 shows a research budget for a project that is planned to take one year to conduct. The major types of resources are broken down as:

Direct Costs

Personnel	Consultants
Professional	Facilities
Staff	Subcontracted services
Equipment	Travel
Supplies	Printing/Publication

Indirect Costs

It is advised by many research funding agencies — whether it be government, private industry or a foundation — that you should include itemized estimates of the approximate cost of personnel time, facilities, supplies or any other contribution to the project. Accordingly, notice in the budget that there is personnel time allocated to the project for which funds are not sought from the granting agency. Also notice that the budget has two total costs calculated: total direct costs and total indirect costs. The indirect costs are usually calculated quite simply as a prearranged percentage of total costs. In the example budget shown here, the indirect costs are 75% of direct personnel, consultant and travel costs.

BUDGET

Direct Costs

Personnel		Effort on Project			Request
Name	Position	% Time	Salary	Fringe	Total
C.D. Williams	Principal Investigator	25	15,000	3,000	—
D.G. Bruce	Co-investigator	15	10,000	2,000	12,000
C.B. James	Statistician	10	3,000	600	3,600
M.G. Coleman	Research Assistant	33	6,000	1,200	7,200
G.L. Bucher	Programmer	25	7,000	1,400	8,400
D.L. Kilhefner	Secretary	50	9,000	1,800	10,800
Subtotals			**$50,000**	**$10,000**	**$42,000**
Consultants: R.V. Roentgen — five (5) days at $300/day					$1,500
Equipment: One (1) personal computer (specify)					$3,500
Supplies: Postage — $50/month — $600 Office supplies — $2,500 Telephone — $100/month for 12 months = $1,200 Copying — $600					$4,900
Facilities: Rental — $1,200/month for 12 months — $14,400 Renovation — $3,500 for office partitions					$17,900
Travel: Local travel for data collection — $50/month Two (2) national meetings/year for two investigators @ $750/trip					$3,000
Subcontracted Service: Printing/publications — $1,700 Computing expenses — $2,600					$4,300
TOTAL DIRECT COSTS					**$77,100**
Total Indirect Costs (overhead): 75% of Personnel, Consultants and Travel					$34,875
TOTAL					**$111,975**

Budget Justification:

Personnel: C.D. Williams will serve as Principal Investigator of the project and will devote 25% of her time overseeing all phases of the grant administration and report writing.

D.G. Bruce is co-investigator for the project and will coordinate all staff activities for the project and be responsible for the calibration of all measures and collection of data.

C.B. James will be responsible for all data analysis and ensure proper programming and use of computer facilities.*

Consultants: R.V. Roentgen is Professor of Radiology at State University and will oversee the standardization and calibration of examiners in diagnostic methods.

Equipment: Personal computer keyboard, CRT console, 256K memory, and letter quality printer.

Facilities: 400 square feet of office space at $3/sq. ft. per month; requires minor renovations for efficient use.

Travel: Local travel is for data collection. Out of state travel is for the principal investigator and co-investigator to attend two national research meetings per year.

Subcontracts: Printing and binding is for 300 copies of the final report. Computing for the major data set is subcontracted to the central computing facility of the university.

---

*Research assistant, programmer and secretary activities should be described only if their responsibilities are out of the ordinary.

Problem 2:
Before going on to the check list for evaluating research proposals, see if you can list the seven primary sections of a research protocol.

1.

2.

3.

4.

5.

6.

7.

EVALUATING RESEARCH PROTOCOLS

Hold it, you're not finished! The first thing to do now that a complete draft of your protocol has been written is to evaluate it yourself. The following check list has been adapted from Blandford et al. These questions can be used to assure that you have not overlooked any of the major questions that a reviewer for a granting agency will probably ask.

1. *Background and Problem*

_____ Is the background information sufficient and is the problem clearly defined?

_____ Has the relevant literature been critically reviewed?

_____ Does the review of the literature support the contention that the answers to the research questions being asked are not already known?

_____ Will the study results be a significant contribution to the scientific area of inquiry?

2. *Objectives and Hypotheses*

_____ Are the objectives or hypotheses stated clearly, and are they defined and derived directly from the statement of the problem?

_____ Are the objectives or hypotheses attainable with the resources available or planned for the project?

_____ Do the objectives or hypotheses clearly indicate the type of data that will need to be collected?

_____ Are assumptions relating to the objectives or hypotheses of the research made explicit?

3. *Research Design*

_____ Are the experimental or survey procedures specified in detail?

_____ If sampling is to be used, is the sampling methodology fully described?

_____ If sampling is to be used, is the population identified fully described?

_____ If sampling is to be used, is the sample size adequate?

_____ If the design is an experiment, is the plan for assignment to control and experimental groups feasible?

_____ If a randomly assigned control group is not planned, will the identification of the comparison groups control the critical variables under study?

_____ What are the limitations of the proposed design?

4. *Data to be Collected*

_____ Have all of the data to be collected been specified?

_____ Are human subjects' considerations satisfied?

_____ Are the data to be collected directly related to the objectives or hypotheses?

_____ Are the measurement procedures (operational definitions) specified in detail?

_____ Are the measurement procedures documented as reliable?

_____ Have the measurement procedures been documented as valid operational definitions of the concepts?

_____ Are the data to be collected in the form needed for testing the hypotheses or achieving the objectives?

5. *Data Analysis and Reporting*

_____ Is the plan for statistical analysis clearly described?

_____ Are the statistical procedures appropriate?

_____ Are computer programs available and accessible to conduct the statistical analyses?

_____ Have adequate pretests of procedures or measurement methods been made or planned?

6. *Work Schedule*

_____ Does the work schedule include all of the major sections of the project?

_____ Is the schedule realistic in view of other commitments and responsibilities of the investigator(s)?

_____ Is the work flow technically logical?

_____ Is the time frame for the project feasible?

7. *Budget and Budget Justification*

_____ Are the number and qualifications of personnel appropriate for the study?

_____ Is the investigator planning to use technical assistance and consultation when necessary?

_____ Will available or planned facilities, equipment and other resources be adequate for this research project?

_____ Have the necessary steps been initiated to secure the cooperative support and agreement by others to participate in the project or provide necessary support?

_____ Does the budget justification address questions about the requested funds that need further explanation?

_____ Are budget items excessive or insufficient or unrelated to the research project?

_____ Do the potential benefits of the study warrant the requested funds?

REVIEW

1) A research protocol is used to tell the *why, what,* and *how* of a research project and the *so what* of the expected results.

2) In evaluating a scientific article ask:
   - What do the authors say?
   - How do they know? and
   - So what?

3) The major sections of a research protocol are:
   - Background and Problem
   - Objectives and Hypotheses
   - Research Design
   - Data to be Collected
   - Data Analysis and Reporting
   - Work Schedule
   - Budget and Budget Justification

4) *Objectives* are usually written when the research project is descriptive or exploratory, while *hypotheses* are usually written when the research project attempts to identify the causal relationships among the study variables.

5) Naming the element, substance or phenomenon to be studied is called the *conceptual definition*. Describing how each element, substance, or phenomenon will be measured in a study is called the *operational definition*.

6) *Survey research* designs select samples from a known population for study. Facts obtained from the sample are generalized to the population from which it was drawn. *Experimental research* randomly assigns or matches the elements, substances, or phenomena under study into experimental and control groups which are then considered to be similar except for the object of the investigation.

7) The protocol should explicitly describe the *data collection* and *data analysis* procedures. This description should include plans for pretesting, training, data processing, statistical analysis, interpretation, and report writing.

8) The administrative components of the research protocol are found in the *budget, budget justification,* and *work schedule.*

SOLUTIONS

Problem 1

The research protocol is used to tell:

1) *why* the research is used;
2) *what* procedures must be conducted;
3. *how* these procedures will be carried out; and
4) *what* results you expect.

Problem 2

1) Background and Problem
2) Objectives and Hypotheses
3) Research Design
4) Data to be Collected
5) Data Analysis and Reporting
6) Work Schedule
7) Budget and Budget Justification

Reference: Blandford, D.H.; Campbell, E.M.; and Warren, G.B. 1984. Introduction to research planning. *Journal of Dental Education* 48:246-250 and 298-301.

POSTTEST 20

Over the past two years in your clinical practice you have noticed that in treating patients with moderate (type II) periodontal disease, you seem to be able to obtain similar clinical results with either non-surgical conservative treatment on some patients or surgical treatment on others. You believe that you might be providing the surgical treatment on the somewhat more difficult cases but you are not sure because you tend to be influenced in these treatment decisions by the patients' fear of surgery or desire to have the surgery because it is covered by insurance.

Write an outline of a research protocol for a project that is designed to test the effectiveness of surgical versus non-surgical treatment regimens on periodontal disease cases that have the same degree of clinical pathology. Be sure that all of the sections of a research protocol discussed in this chapter are included. Also include a budget and work schedule, but not data collection forms.

Omit details of the research design until after you have completed Chapter 21.

YOUR ANSWERS
TO POSTTEST 20

Name:

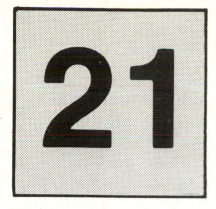

CHAPTER 21

CLINICAL TRIALS AND EXPERIMENTAL DESIGNS

INTRODUCTION

New dental technologies have expanded the number and types of treatment modalities available to providers and patients. In addition to experience and clinical judgment, more scientifically rigorous information is being sought on which to base the entry of patient care modalities used in dental practice. As a result there is a growing need to evaluate new preventive agents, patient management regimens, and surgical procedures.

Clinical trials provide a scientific approach by which new treatments can be compared with traditional treatments. The conduct of a clinical trial involves the application of a controlled experimental design where the patients in the study population are randomly assigned to treatment and control (e.g., standard care) groups. Two kinds of clinical trials are presented in this chapter. The *randomized clinical trial* (RCT) represents the true experimental design. *Non-randomized clinical trials* use quasi-experimental designs that can be applied practically in many clinical settings. In addition, pre-experimental designs aid in the formulation of study objectives.

OBJECTIVES

1) You will be able to describe the differences between the three major classes of experimental designs.
2) You will understand why a clinical trial research design is a rigorous scientific method for detecting the difference between two treatments if one exists.
3) You will be able to list and discuss the major characteristics of a well-designed clinical trial.

EXPERIMENTAL DESIGNS

The use of sound experimental design provides the fundamental characteristic of a clinical trial. Three classes of experimental designs are briefly described here: 1) true experimental designs; 2) quasi-experimental designs; and 3) pre-experimental designs.

True Experimental Designs

True experimental designs use randomization to assign patients to treatment groups for the purpose of initially equalizing the experimental and control groups, thus the term *randomized clinical trials* (RCT). The two types of true experimental designs which are most often used in clinical trials are 1) the randomized parallel group trial, and 2) the randomized crossover trial.

Randomized Parallel Group Trial:

Campbell and Stanley (1963) described a true experimental design which they denote as a randomized pretest-posttest control group design. This design is identified as the *randomized parallel group trial* here and represents the most frequently used true experimental design. Figure 21.1 outlines this design.

Figure 21.1   **Randomized Parallel Group Trial**

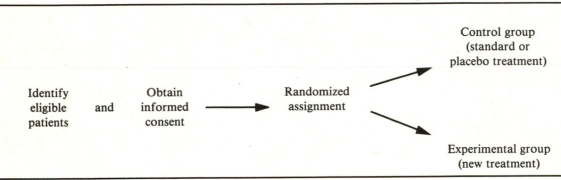

The experimental design for the randomized parallel group trial can be expressed as follows using a modification of the original notation of Campbell and Stanley:

$$\text{Eligible patients with informed consent} \longrightarrow R \underset{0_1 \; X \; 0_2 \quad \text{(Experimental Group)}}{\overset{0_1 \quad 0_2 \quad \text{(Control Group)}}{\lessgtr}}$$

where:

0_1 = measurements of oral health before treatment;
0_2 = measurements of oral health after treatment;
X = receipt of experimental treatment; and
R = random assignment to the control or experimental group.

The most important features of this design are the use of randomization (R) to assign patients to experimental and control groups and the inclusion of pre-treatment or baseline measures (0_1). These feature control for the major alternative hypotheses, or biases, which threaten the interpretation of the clinical trial results. For example, the effect of history (such as a concurrent decline in the incidence of dental caries) is equally active within the control and experimental groups; this effect can be eliminated by means of a comparison of before and after differences (0_1–0_2) between study groups. Similarly, individual biological differences among patients are controlled by the randomization procedure which is a uniquely unbiased mechanism for assigning patients to treatments.

This design can be extended to include three or more treatments; in some trials both a standard treatment and a placebo are included as "control" groups with a three treatment randomized parallel group design. Further improvements are accomplished through the inclusion of multiple pre-treatment measures to establish baseline trends, and the inclusion of multiple post-treatment measures to establish evidence regarding efficacy and safety over time. These modifications lead to what is commonly referred to as a repeated measures design.

The randomized parallel group trial design has been used to evaluate clinical dental procedures in the comparison of surgical versus non-surgical periodontal therapy. After an initial prophylaxis and oral hygiene phase, patients (or different quadrants within the same patients) with equal periodontal disease severity as measured by calibrated clinical examiners are randomly assigned to receive surgical treatment from a periodontist or deep scaling and root planing from a dental hygienist. Post operative measurements of attachment level, bone loss, mobility, calculus, pocket depth, gingivitis, and plaque are taken at periodic intervals by the same examiners who are blind to which patients or quadrants have received which treatment. A clinical trial that used the randomized parallel group design has been reported by Rundle et al. (1985).

Randomized Crossover Trial

A second commonly used true experimental design in clinical trials is the *randomized crossover trial*. This design only applies to diseases or physical conditions that are palliative rather than curative, and which, therefore, recur when medication or treatment is withheld. In particular, crossover designs are often applied to chronic conditions, such as chronic recurring gingivitis, where outcome is measured in terms of short term relief of signs and symptoms. The design is represented in Figure 21.2.

Figure 21.2   **Randomized Crossover Trial**

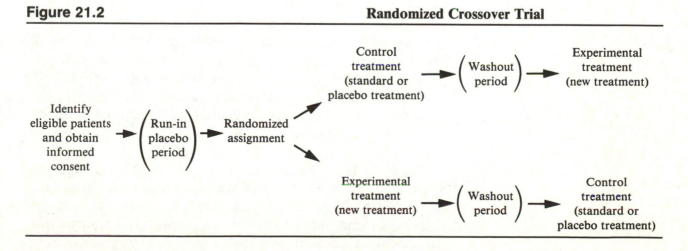

There are several design features of the randomized crossover clinical trial that are important to recognize. First, a pre-randomization *run-in* period is usually required. During this period the patient commonly receives a "placebo" treatment, such as standard prophylaxis and oral hygiene instruction, and the condition of the entire study sample is monitored until the physiological condition of each patient has reached a stable baseline. At that point each patient who continues to meet the eligibility criteria is randomly assigned to alternative sequence groups — one sequence consisting of the new treatment followed by the standard treatment, the other consisting of the standard treatment followed by the new treatment. Hence, each patient is scheduled to receive a *sequence* of both the experimental and control treatments, but in opposite orders, thus signifying the crossover character of this particular clinical trial design.

A second important feature of this design is that a *wash-out* period is needed after the first treatment has been stopped in order to allow each patient's physiological condition to return to its baseline levels. This wash-out period should be long enough so that the therapeutic effect of the first treatment does not carry over into the second treatment time period. If this precaution is not taken, a carry-over effect may distort the results of the study.

The crossover trial has the same benefits of randomization that a parallel group trial possesses. In addition, this design has the advantage of providing more precise comparisons of treatments through the use of each patient as his/her own control; this feature reduces between-patient variability and generally results in a need for fewer patients to be studied than would be required in a parallel group trial. The fact that each patient receives both treatments is often viewed as a benefit for ethical reasons as well, since no patient is denied the new therapy or procedure.

The randomized crossover trial is most commonly used in dentistry to study the effects of agents that improve poor oral hygiene which is known to be a reversible condition. During the run-in placebo period all patients receive a similar "standard" oral hygiene regimen and baseline measures are obtained. Patients are then randomized to a sequence in which they receive the new oral hygiene regimen followed by the standard oral hygiene regimen, or vice versa. The wash-out period between the two treatment periods must be long enough to allow the oral hygiene condition to return to its baseline level before the second treatment period is started. This design has been used to test the effectiveness of mouth rinses, denture cleansers, toothpastes and other oral hygiene aids.

Crossover studies are a form of repeated measures designs and can be extended to three or more treatment/sequence groups as long as sufficient wash-out periods are used. However, the complexity of the analysis increases with the number of treatments to be compared. Further discussion of crossover trials is presented by Pocock (1983).

Problem 1:

What is the major characteristic of the disease or conditon being treated that would make it amenable to a randomized crossover trial?

Your Solution:

Quasi-Experimental Designs

Whenever possible the design of a clinical trial should include a randomized control group. Trials which are not based on such designs may be subject to threats to validity which can compromise the strength of conclusions. However, it is sometimes not feasible to employ a true experimental design in every clinical investigation. In carrying out post-marketing surveillance of the long-term safety of a drug patients are not usually randomly allocated to treatment groups. Instead, observations of adverse effects can be assessed using classical epidemiological designs such as the case/control or cohort methodology. These methods, which are described in most epidemiologic texts (see Kleinbaum, Kupper and Morganstern, 1982), are essentially applications of quasi-experimental designs.

Other types of studies where true experimental designs cannot be applied are health services or other public policy evaluations where large populations or whole communities are to be compared. In such instances, some control of threats to validity can be achieved by means of quasi-experimental designs. These designs are described in detail by Campbell and Stanley (1963) and more recently by Cook and Campbell (1979). Two quasi-experimental designs are briefly described below.

Non-Equivalent Control Group Design

A quasi-experimental design which is quite similar to the randomized parallel group trial has been denoted by Campbell and Stanley as the *non-equivalent control group design*. This design may be identified in modified form as follows:

$$\frac{M \ 0_1 \qquad 0_2}{M \ 0_1 \ X \ 0_2}$$
Control Group

Experimental Group

where,

0_1 = measurements of the disease before treatment;

0_2 = measurements of the disease after treatment;

X = receipt of experimental treatment; and

M = a matching procedure for control and experimental groups based on demographic, behavioral and physiological variables that might represent alternative hypotheses for interpreting the differences between the two groups.

Note the similarity of this design notation to the randomized parallel group design; the one very important difference being the lack of randomization.

The non-equivalent control group design is applicable when a treatment is to be evaluated by collecting data before and after the treatment is applied, but randomization is not possible. In large community studies the "treatment" may represent a change in health policy and it may be impractical to assign subjects, families or clinics to treatments at random. If a control group is not included, then it is not possible to determine whether observed changes are due to the treatment or due to factors such as the particular selection characteristics of patients included and history effects, i.e., other changes in the community outside the control of the study. When randomization is not possible, then some control of selection effects or other biases resulting from follow-up over time can be achieved through the choice of a similar but non-randomized control group. In a large population study the control group can be a neighboring community; in a hospital study it can be another carefully chosen ward or service. The "non-equivalent" group is chosen so as to match the study group as closely as possible on all of the important characteristics that could make a difference in the outcome measures. Differences between groups at the end of the study can then be inferred to be related to the receipt of the experimental treatment. Simultaneous comparisons over time in the study and control groups provide improved estimates of efficacy and safety since changes which are not due to the study treatment should affect both groups.

A classic example of the application of this design was the Newburgh-Kingston Caries-Fluoride Study. In 1945, two cities, Newburgh and Kingston, New York, which are located about 35 miles apart, agreed to participate in a study of the effectiveness of fluoride on the prevention of dental caries. Fluoride was added to the water supply of Newburgh, while no change in the water supply was made for Kingston. The efficacy of fluoridated water in preventing dental caries was clearly shown in this study. (See Ast et al., 1956.)

Two Group Matched Time Series

Further improvements can be achieved over the non-equivalent control group design by collecting pre-treatment and post-treatment data at several points in time. In a manner similar to the repeated measures randomized parallel group design, time series data allow for estimates of trends before and after treatment.

This design is represented as follows:

$$\frac{M \; 0_1 \; 0_2 \; 0_3 \; 0_4 \; X \; 0_5 \; 0_6 \; 0_7 \; 0_8}{M \; 0_1 \; 0_2 \; 0_3 \; 0_4 \quad\;\; 0_5 \; 0_6 \; 0_7 \; 0_8}.$$

A strength of the design is provided by the repeated measures which give a more stable long term view of the patients under study. For example, an immediate short term effect of the treatment (X) could appear as an improvement in the patients' condition between 0_4 and 0_5. However, the 0_1, 0_2, and 0_3 measures before the treatment, and the 0_6, 0_7, and 0_8 measures after the treatment now contribute to a time series of eight measures from which any 0_4-0_5 changes can be interpreted more appropriately. Because of the ability to match patients between the two groups and follow patients over long run-in and follow-up periods, this design represents the most favorable of the quasi-experimental designs as regards helping to infer cause and effect relationships.

In summary, the *non-equivalent control group design* and *two group matched time series design* are two examples of many quasi-experimental designs which may be possible depending on the setting of the study to be conducted. The two primary strategies to minimize threats to validity which may be present due to the lack of randomization are the use of matching to enhance comparability between treatment and (non-equivalent) control groups, and the use of repeated measures both pre and post treatment in order to assess trends over time.

Problem 2:

What are the key features of the quasi-experimental designs outlined above that enhance their ability to provide scientific information?

Your Solution:

Pre-Experimental Designs

The final group of designs for clinical trials is not, in fact, either true or quasi-experimental. They are therefore weak in their ability to provide scientifically valid results that causally relate the treatment to the outcome measures.

Case Study

Frequently, clinical information is presented in the form of a *case study* on a group of patients in order to imply cause and effect relationships between treatment and outcome. A single group of dental patients that receives treatment and then is followed for effects provides no chance to compare the result of treatment with another group of similar patients. Moreover, a case study series is often reported as an after-thought and often does not even have the ability to provide before measures on the same patients. *The documentation of individual patient experiences is, however, a method for generating ideas and exploring possibilities that should be studied.* An example of the use of case studies in making cause and effect inferences can be found in the 1985 emergence of the relationship between smokeless tobacco and oral cancer.

Panel Study or One Group Pretest-Posttest

The *panel study or one group pretest-posttest design* is mentioned here as a second example of the kinds of non-scientific research design to avoid when conducting clinical trial investigations. In this design one group of patients is measured at baseline and then followed through therapy and beyond. Threats to validity include the effect of history and concurrent events, aging and maturation of patients, and a statistical regression effect in which the highest (or lowest) measures on the pretest have a natural tendency to move down (or up) on the posttest because that was the only direction in which any change could occur.

Problem 3:

Identify an appropriate clinical trial design for a clinical question of your choice and explain why the design you chose is appropriate.

Your Solution:

CHARACTERISTICS OF CLINICAL TRIALS

There are four stages in the implementation of a clinical trial: (1) specifying the research protocol, (2) collecting the data, (3) analyzing the results, and (4) writing the final report. In writing the research protocol, the investigator details the research design. The design decisions are then implemented through carefully monitored "data collection" and "statistical analysis" procedures. Finally, the results of the trial are communicated through a written report. This section discusses the characteristics of these stages and the *strengthening measures* that are important to consider during the implementation of clinical trials. The strengthening measures are summarized as headings in the margin of what follows.

Problem 4:

What are the four main stages in conducting a clinical trial?

Your Solution:

THE RESEARCH PROTOCOL

In describing a clinical trial it is necessary to apply the first three sections of the research protocol — Background and Problem, Objectives, and Research Design. Given an understanding of the problem, the specific tasks incorporated into the research protocol are defining the study objectives, deciding upon the research design, identifying and selecting appropriate patients, obtaining informed consent to participate in the study, randomizing patients into study groups, and specifying the sample size. All design-related issues should be summarized in a research protocol which clearly describes each of these issues and states how they are to be addressed throughout the duration of the study. The details of a research protocol have been discussed in Chapter 20; this chapter now focuses on the use of a research protocol in implementing a clinical trial.

Defining Study Objectives

The preliminary step to carrying out a clinical trial is to define the objectives of the trial. For example, is the trial intended to assess dose tolerance, i.e., the highest dose which can be administered before the onset of side effects, or is it intended to assess the comparative effectiveness of a therapy? As emphasized in Chapter 20 the objectives should also include a clear statement of the major hypotheses to be investigated and the measures to be collected and analyzed in order to test these hypotheses.

Given a statement of study objectives, the following design issues must be specified in the third section of the protocol:

1) The type of research design to be employed (e.g., parallel group, crossover, quasi-experimental, etc.);
2) the experimental and control treatments to be compared;
3) the preventive, diagnostic or therapeutic regimen to be evaluated;
4) the clinical outcome criteria that provide the basis for the evaluation.

Eligibility Criteria

In order that the search for the appropriate patient population can be efficient, clear inclusion criteria must be written so that the health care professionals responsible for conducting the study can identify potential participants without wasted effort.

The eligibility criteria should be spelled out explicitly in the research protocol to include:

1) physiological measures of the disease or condition to be treated;
2) probable sources of patients (these should assure that the study sample is as representative of the population as is feasible);
3) diagnostic criteria for confirmation of each disease level;
4) appropriate absence of other confounding conditions; and
5) appropriate medical history for allowing evaluation of the treatment under study.

Some flexibility is apparent in these criteria because certain criteria may be too strict for one particular trial, while another may be too flexible in admitting inappropriate patients. In general, however, the decision rules for inclusion or exclusion of each patient should be clear for the specific clinical trial being conducted.

Data Collection Forms

Clinical trial data are often collected on special forms designed for the particular trial under consideration. The types of data usually collected are summarized in the data collection section. Consideration should be given to the methods of processing the data since they will influence the layout and coding of data collection forms. Data processing requirements must then be balanced against the conditions under which the forms will be completed. For example, a data processor may prefer a numerical quantity to be entered in a box for ease of data entry, but a busy dental auxilliary who is completing the forms may prefer to check one or more items from a list.

Informed Consent

Obtaining a legally sound informed consent is an absolute necessity in every clinical trial. This consent must be in writing and be signed by the patient or guardian. The consent statement should include the following items:

1) description of the condition being treated;
2) description of treatment options;
3) explanation of the procedure for assigning each patient to the experimental or standard treatment; and
4) description of the possible side effects of each treatment group.

Some of the ethical issues related to obtaining informed consent are discussed in the final section of this chapter.

Random Assignment

As previously noted, the use of statistical randomization procedures to allocate patients to treatment groups is a key component of any true experimental design. The primary purpose of random allocation is to guard against any systematic bias in the assignment of patients to either the standard or experimental treatment. In regard to the statistical analysis, randomization is intended to insure the homogeneity of the comparison groups prior to the initiation of therapy. This homogeneity in turn improves the validity of conclusions drawn from post-treatment comparisons of efficacy measures.

The basic concept of all randomization schemes is that each patient is equally likely to be assigned either the standard or experimental treatment. The procedures for carrying out randomization vary depending on the type of study design being used. However, in their simplest form, randomization procedures simulate tossing a coin for each patient to decide which treatment is to be received. In actuality, these procedures usually are carried out using computer generated random number listings.

Sample Size Considerations

The design of a clinical trial should also include a specification of the sample size, i.e., the number of patients to be treated in each group. The sample size needs to be sufficiently large to yield reproducible findings.

To determine how large is "large" in any clinical trial, the following issues should be considered.

1) *Clinical Issues:* The investigators must first determine how large a treatment difference is clinically important and therefore should be detected by the trial. For example, in a periodontal disease study, does the investigator want the trial to be able to detect a 1mm or 2mm difference in pocket depth or attachment level between the surgery and the nonsurgery patients? This is strictly a clinical decision, and the clinicians should decide what really makes a difference. Generally, the larger the clinical difference to be detected, the smaller the sample size needed.

   A second clinical issue is the ethical problem of how many patients are to be denied a new treatment (i.e., subjected to a placebo) or subjected to a new experimental treatment which is yet unproven. The denial of fluorides to control groups is raised as an ethical problem in current day preventive dentistry trials. There is no simple rule to guide clinicians in this area, except: "above all else, do no harm."

2) *Statistical Issues:* The primary statistical issue related to sample size is the level of confidence desired about final estimates of safety and efficacy and the power of the statistical tests to be performed. This concept is tied directly to the amount of variability in the key measures of interest. In order to improve the confidence level in final estimates for a given level of power, a large sample size is required. As the variability in response measures increases a larger sample size is needed to achieve a desired confidence level.

   Another statistical issue related to sample size is the concept of balance in assigning numbers of patients to treatment groups. For most common designs maximum power is achieved by assigning equal numbers of patients to each treatment group. However, there are some special instances where, due to ethical or other non-statistical reasons, unequal samples are chosen for each treatment. Specific formulas for determining sample size for clinical trials and a more complete discussion of these issues are presented by Pocock (1983).

Problem 5:

Before going on to Data Collection try this practice exercise in formulating clinical research questions:

a. Describe in general terms three dental procedures which can be assessed by means of clinical trials. Try to think of a preventive, a diagnostic, and a theraputic regimen.

b. Identify the types of patient who would benefit from each of these procedures and the sources of patients who could be chosen for inclusion in the study.

c. In each case identify the standard therapy, if any, which currently exists and the feasibility of using this therapy as a comparative treatment in a randomized clinical trial.

Your Solution:

DATA COLLECTION

All data collected for each study patient should be included on a separate case report form; the design of this form and the definition of all variables should be decided upon prior to the initiation of the study. Complete directions must be provided in the protocol as to how and when each section of the case report form is to be filled out. In most cases, data are entered by the clinical investigator in order to insure highest quality; however, in some studies patients may directly record findings on patient self-report forms. In either case, specific procedures to insure the validity and reliability of all data should be included in both the collection and processing stages of the study.

Adherence and Compliance

Adherence by investigators and project managers to protocol conditions for the treatment and control groups should be monitored. The procedures for conducting the study must explicitly guard against contamination among the groups under study. Similarly, the *compliance of patients* to their assigned regimens should be monitored. Deviations from adherence to the study protocol by investigators or from compliance with treatment regimens by patients must be recorded and considered in the evaluation of results.

Double Blind

An important procedure that is a standard feature of clinical trials is the collection of data in a double blind fashion. Patients should be unable to determine whether they are in the treatment or the control group, i.e. blind to their assigned group. In addition, the clinicians who collect the data should be unable to determine which patients are receiving the new versus the standard treatment method. Fulfillment of these two conditions constitutes the *double blind* design that helps to insure the validity and reliability of data collection procedures.

Treatment Complications

Another procedure that will aid in the analyses and final interpretation is the recording of *treatment complications*. Decision rules should be written into the study protocol which allow the treatment regimen of a patient to be discontinued based on adverse reactions or worsening of patient's condition. The classifying of complications and recording the cases lost to follow up will provide data that may be important to the interpretation of the study.

Operational Definition of Outcome

It is most important to provide clear *operational definitions* of the primary clinical outcomes of the study. Then, detailed measurement procedures must be documented. For example, in a trial of periodontal disease treatment the primary clinical outcome might be the gingival attachment level. An operational definition of this outcome is millimeters of improvement or loss of the attachment level. Actual measurement is obtained with a calibrated periodontal probe (see cover) using the cemento-enamel junction as the reference point.

In addition to the key clinical outcomes, several other types of data are collected in most trials. Usually, these data serve to provide background on the types of patients studied and details of the clinical experience gained during the trial. There are five general types of data collected in most clinical trials:

1) Pre-treatment: These data include demographic and background characteristics of study patients together with relevant medical history information.

2) Efficacy: These data should include specific measures of treatment effectiveness which are derived directly from the study objectives and specific hypotheses to be tested. In addition to assessments by the clinical investigators, patient assessments are also useful in some studies. For most key efficacy measures it is important to collect data immediately prior to the initiation of therapy (baseline) at each treatment visit and then again at the end of therapy.

3) Safety: A systematic mechanism for assessing and recording all side effects or adverse events must be included in the data procedures of any clinical trial. In addition, pre- and post-treatment measures of vital signs, laboratory evaluations and physical examinations are needed to assess patient safety over the course of the study.

4) Concomitant events: Provision must be made for recording treatment modifications, compliance, and other concomitant therapies. Life style features such as smoking, caffeine consumption, alcohol, and exercise may be monitored.

5) Administrative data: These data include patient identification, randomization codes, treatment labels, dropout status and reason for dropout, a study completion form that records which types of patient data have been completed and which are missing, and tracking information to document patient recruitment and trial progress.

ANALYSIS

The fundamental consideration in the analysis of clinical trials is that the results of the analysis are 1) credible, 2) capable of being reproduced, and 3) if replicate studies were undertaken, the results would be similar. Thus, the analysis of a clinical trial provides an accurate summary of data obtained on groups of patients who are equivalent in essentially all respects other than the receipt of the treatment, and whose response to the treatment is representative of some large set of patients with a similar disease or condition.

The analysis methods used should be specifically directed at the objectives and hypotheses stated in the study protocol; the primary statistical methods should be outlined prior to data collection. Additional methods can be applied if the initial data analysis suggests their appropriateness.

Reported Statistics

The specific measures which should be summarized in a statistical analysis are:

1) patient demographic and pre-treatment characteristics to demonstrate baseline homogeneity of treatment groups;
2) descriptions of inconsistencies in study procedures, protocol violations, and patterns of incomplete data;
3) response variables pertaining to the efficacy of the treatment;
4) results of laboratory tests and physical exams pertaining to a variety of physiologic measurements to note changes which may be related to the assessment of safety;
5) descriptions of side effects (or adverse experiences) and their possible relationships with treatment; and
6) results for patient subgroups that are of clinical importance (e.g. severe patients).

A useful approach to determining the appropriate statistical methods is to classify the clinical outcome measures according to three types.

(i) Dichotomous (e.g. healed vs not healed), or more generally nominal if there are several categories; in this case X^2 is an appropriate analysis strategy.
(ii) Ordinal (e.g. classifications of improvement as worse, no change, slight, moderate, completely healed); here, nonparametric methods using ranks are generally appropriate.
(iii) Continuous (e.g. blood pressure determinations); t-tests and ANOVA are usually appropriate for these type of data.

A fourth type of data that has not been discussed in this book is survival data. Here, time until a critical event such as death is collected. The complication arises that some patients are likely to be lost to follow-up and so the statistical problem of censoring of survival time data has to be dealt with. Techniques for survival data that account for censoring are discussed by Pocock (1983).

REPORT WRITING

The main purpose of a written report of a clinical trial is to summarize the findings of the trial in an objective manner so that the outcome can be brought to the attention of the scientific community. The basic outline of a report was presented in the previous chapter. In many cases reporting is accomplished in dental or other scientific journals. The report of a clinical trial should be written in sufficient detail to allow other investigators to:

1) accept or reject your conclusions based on the data presented in the report; and
2) replicate the study.

Concise Reporting

Writing for the scientific community requires precision, clarity, and conciseness. Your writing should reflect a logical understanding of your findings in a style which communicates those findings coherently. A scientific writing style includes careful attention to word choice and relatively short, to-the-point sentences. Uncomplicated, simple sentences will communicate your ideas most clearly. You may choose to begin by identifying a concept, then elaborating the idea, and then restating or generalizing the original concept. Above all else, leave time between writing drafts to let your ideas "settle." Then go back to the report to revise carefully and objectively, keeping in mind stylistic requirements as well as scientific accuracy.

Generalizability

One of the issues that will be raised by a critical reader is that of generalizability. The question of generalizability is: To what extent are the results of a particular clinical trial applicable to other patient populations who have the same disease or condition? This is an issue because the patients who participated in the trial were not drawn from a pool of all patients for whom the newly developed treatment might seem to be appropriate. One of the methods for improving generalizability is the use of large multi-investigator trials. Typically in these studies generalizability is assessed through comparisons of efficacy findings between investigators and between patient subgroups. The consistency of results across investigators and patient subgroups helps to confirm the generalizability of findings from a particular trial.

In reading a report, you must decide whether the results can be applied to your patients. Three considerations are appropriate in making this judgment.

1) Does the clinical trial encompass the entire range of patients to whom the results may be generalized?
2) Are there replicate studies by other investigators with similar findings?
3) Do the clinical trial results demonstrate that treatment differences are homogeneous across investigators and across different levels of patient demographic and pre-treatment characteristics?

If these three questions can be answered in the affirmative, the generalizability of the clinical trial results in question is enhanced.

ETHICAL ISSUES

In every clinical trial special attention should be paid to ethical considerations and, in particular, to whether it is ethically acceptable for patients to participate in the trial. In designing a trial you need to be keenly aware of the balance between patient care and scientific progress.

A detailed discussion of ethical considerations is provided by Pocock (1983). For the purposes of this text it is sufficient to point out four key areas where ethics need to be considered when designing a clinical trial.

1) Double-blind trials — In most cases neither the investigator nor the patient knows which treatment is being received; this is intended to avoid possible sources of bias. However, the protocol should include procedures which will allow the investigator to identify which treatment a patient is receiving so that in the event a severe adverse reaction occurs, this information can be used in treating the complication. In most pharmaceutical trials the use of "peel-off" labels on medication serves to address this issue.

2) Placebo controls — In many clinical trials the control treatment is a placebo. This procedure allows the statistician to estimate the true treatment effects by adjusting for placebo effects. An important question is raised regarding the ethics of "treating" diseased patients with a placebo. Some solutions to this problem can be achieved through special design features. For example, a randomized crossover design where all patients receive standard therapy for at least some time interval can be used. Also, a follow-up period in which all patients get crossed over to the standard treatment can be inlcuded.

3) Patient consent — As mentioned earlier, written informed consent must be obtained from every patient participating in a clinical trial. The standards that govern this consent are legal requirements in the United States. Most consent forms are signed before the randomization procedure takes place but this chronology is not a necessary requirement.

4) IRB — An Institutional Review Board oversees and evaluates research protocols, considering both ethical and scientific questions. This review process is performed independently of the clinical trial investigator and, consequently, provides an objective checking system for the study.

In summary, ethical issues are important to consider both in the design and in the specification of the method of conduct of the trial. A formal consideration of the ethical issues involved in each study can have a great influence on whether or not the trial can or should be conducted at all.

Problem 6:

What are the major characteristics that strengthen a well conducted clinical trial?

Your Solution:

REVIEW

1) There are two major types of clinical trials that use true experimental designs; 1) the randomized parallel group trial, and 2) the randomized crossover trial.

2) Two quasi-experimental designs described in this chapter are 1) the non-equivalent control group design, and 2) the two group matched time series. These designs use matching and trends over time as key features of their designs.

3) Pre-experimental designs such as case studies or panel studies have very limited scientific ability to determine cause and effect relationships. These descriptive studies are appropriate only for generating ideas and developing hypotheses that can be tested with other study designs.

4) The four main stages in planning and conducting a clinical trial are: 1) the research protocol 2) data collection 3) analysis and 4) report writing.

5) The major characteristics that strengthen a well conducted study are listed in the solution to problem 6 below.

SOLUTIONS

Problem 1:

The disease or condition will recur when the treatment regimen is withheld.

Problem 2:

Quasi-experimental designs attempt to 1) match the patients in the control and experimental groups, and/or 2) measure the trend of the effects over time to improve their scientific validity.

Problem 3:

There is no single answer to the problem. Explain your choice of one of the two true experimental designs, or three Quasi-experimental designs. One key question is whether you can randomly assign patients. Alternatively, you will have to use a matching procedure.

Problem 4:

The four main stages in conducting a clinical trial are: 1) the research protocol, 2) data collection, 3) analysis and 4) report writing.

Problem 5:

There is no single answer to this problem. Preventive, diagnostic and therapeutic services on which clinical trials could be conducted tend to be either relatively new or procedures for which there is as yet no scientific basis. Attempting to distinguish the types of patients who could benefit from the service, identifying the patient who could be chosen for inclusion in the study, and describing the standard or comparative treatment for the control group will be instructive for you. An example of a possible answer is:

a) Services amenable to evaluation by clinic trials;
   1) Sealants
   2) Periodic vertical anterior bitewing radiographs
   3) Extraction of asymptomatic impacted third molars.

b) Types and sources of eligible patients;
   1) Children aged seven and 12 years, found in local elementary schools
   2) Older adult patients, found in Veterans Administration ambulatory dental service programs
   3) Twenty-year-olds, found in higher education institutions.

c) Standard therapy used as comparative procedure.
   1) Topical fluoride or no preventive service
   2) Anterior periapical radiographs
   3) No treatment

Problem 6:

The Research Protocol
   1) Study objectives are defined.
   2) There are clear eligibility criteria for selection and rejection of patients.
   3) Well designed data collection forms are available.
   4) Appropriate informed consent has been obtained.

5) Patients are randomly assigned to study groups by an unbiased procedure, otherwise careful matching has occurred where randomization is not possible.

6) The sample size provides sufficient statistical power and the desired level of confidence.

Data Collection

7) The treatment and control procedures are completely described, and the criteria for adherence and compliance have been provided. Data assurring that protocol violations are minimal are available.

8) Double blind conditions have been maintained during data collection.

9) Treatment complications are recorded.

10) The operational definitions of all outcome or response measures are clear.

Analysis

11) The reported statistics rely on data analyses and statistical methods that are appropriate for the type of data and measurement scales that have been used.

Report Writing

12) The written report is concise and provides sufficient details to a) accept or reject the stated conclusion based on the data presented in the report, and b) replicate the study.

13) The generalizability of study results has been considered.

Ethics

14) Ethical issues appear to have guided the design and conduct of the trial.

POSTTEST 21

Identify a clinical condition and design a study for which a two group matched time series design is appropriate. Tell how each of the major characteristics of a well-designed clinical trial is addressed by your study.

REFERENCES

1) Ast, D.B., Smith, D.J. Wachs, B. and Cantwell, K.T., Newburgh-Kingston Caries-Fluoride Study XIV. Findings after 10 years of experience. *J. Am. Dent. Assoc.* 52:314-325, 1956.

2) Campbell, D.T. and Stanley, J.C. *Experimental and Quasi-Experimental Designs for Research.* Chicago: Rand McNally College Publishing Company, 1963.

3) Cook, T.D. and Campbell, D.T. *Quasi-Experimentation: Design and Analysis Issues for Field Settings.* Chicago: Rand McNally College Publishing Company, 1979.

4) Deniston, O.L. and Rosenstock, I.M. The validity of non-experimental designs for evaluating health services. *Health Services Reports* 88(2):153-164, 1973.

5) Kleinbaum, D.G., Kupper, L.L., and Morganstern, H., Epidmiologic Research: Principles and Quantitative Methods. Lifetime Learning Publications, Belmont, Calif. 1982.

6) Pocock, S.J. Clinical Trials, a practical approach. John Wiley and Sons. New York 1983, xii + 266 pp.

7) Rundle, D.; Howell, H.; Jenkin, S.; and Douglass, C. Clinical trial comparing surgical and non-surgical treatment of periodontal disease. *Journal of Dental Research.* 64:1004. March, 1985.

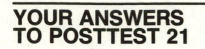

SUGGESTIONS FOR FURTHER READING

Andrews, F.M. et al. *A guide for selecting statistical techniques for analyzing social science data: second edition*. Ann Arbor: Survey Research Center, Institute for Social Research, The University of Michigan, 1981.

Armitage, P. *Statistical methods in medical research*. New York: John Wiley and Sons, 1971.

Blandford, D.H.; Campbell, E.M.; and Warren, G.B. 1984. Introduction to research planning. *Journal of Dental Education* 48:246–250 and 298–301.

Campbell, D.T., and Stanley, J.C. *Experimental and quasi-experimental designs for research*. Chicago: Rand McNally College Publishing Company, 1963.

Colton, T. *Statistics in medicine*. Boston: Little, Brown and Company, 1974.

Cook, T.D., and Stanley, D.T. *Quasi-experimentation: design and analysis issues for field settings*. Chicago: Rand McNally College Publishing Company, 1979.

Draper, N., and Smith, H. *Applied regression analysis: second edition*. New York: John Wiley and Sons, 1982.

Fleiss, J.L. *Statistical methods for rates and proportions: second edition*. New York: John Wiley and Sons, 1981.

Haack, D.G. *Statistical literacy: a guide and interpretation*. North Scituate: Duxbury Press, 1979.

Huitema, B.E. *The analysis of covariance and alternatives*. New York: John Wiley and Sons, 1980.

Kleinbaum, D.G.; Kupper, L.L.: and Morganstern, H. *Epidemiologic research: principles and quantitative methods*. Belmont: Lifetime Learning Publications, 1982.

Koch, G.G., and Sollecito, W.A. 1984. Statistical considerations in the design, analysis, and interpretation of comparative clinical studies. *Drug Information Journal* 18:131–151.

Lehman, E.L. *Nonparametrics: statistical methods based on ranks*. San Francisco: Holden-Day Inc., 1975.

Lentner, C. ed. *Introduction to statistics, statistical tables, mathematical formula* 8th ed. vol. 2 New Jersey: Ciba-Geigy Corporation.

Neter, J.; Wasserman, W.; and Kutner, M.H. *Applied linear statistical models: second edition*. Homewood, Illinois: Richard D. Irwin, Inc., 1985.

Pocock, J. *Clinical trials: a practical approach*. New York: John Wiley and Sons, 1983.

Rosner, B. *Fundamentals of biostatistics*. Boston: Duxbury Press, 1982.

APPENDIX

FREQUENTLY USED DENTAL MEASUREMENTS

The following measures and indices are frequently used in dental research and consequently quoted in the scientific literature. In oral health surveys they are used to quantify and compare the prevalence of dental caries and periodontal diseases in different populations. In clinical trials they are used to compare the effects that specified treatments or interventions have on the oral health of the experimental group or target population as compared to control groups or other comparison populations.

When evaluating any index, measurement, or experimental design, one must consider its *validity* and *reliability*. Validity refers to the appropriateness and accuracy of the chosen methodology in assessing the situation that you are trying to measure. Sensitivity and specificity are ways to assess validity in some types of experimental designs. Reliability refers to the ability of the chosen methodology to be repeated yielding consistent and reproducible results.

THE DMF INDICES

The **Decayed-Missing-or-Filled Index (DMF)** was developed by Klein, Palmer and Knutson during a study of the dental status and dental treatment needs of elementary schoolchildren in Hagerstown, Maryland in 1935. It has become the primary index used in dental studies to quantify the incidence and prevalence of dental caries. The DMF Index gives an indication of both the past and present dental caries experience because it includes a consideration of teeth that have carious lesions as well as teeth that have been treated for dental caries. It can be used as a count of the number of decayed, missing or filled *teeth* per individual **(DMFT)** or a count of the number of decayed, missing or filled tooth *surfaces* per individual **(DMFS).** The numerator is the sum of the number of "D" teeth, "M" teeth and "F" teeth or surfaces. The denominator for this count is the number of individuals examined, and not the total number of teeth examined. When the DMFS Index is used, each of the five tooth surfaces are considered separately.

Criteria have been determined by the Caries Measurement Task Group at the American Dental Association Conference on Clinical

Testing of Cariostatic Agents, the National Caries Program of the National Institute of Dental Research and others as to when to diagnose a tooth as being decayed. It is easy to diagnose a large lesion, but examiners must be calibrated against specific criteria in order to be consistent in their diagnosis of incipient or borderline lesions. A tooth or surface that is both carious and filled is usually counted as carious. A remaining root is counted as 1 carious tooth or 5 carious surfaces.

The "M" portion of the index only considers teeth that are missing due to caries. Teeth that have been extracted for orthodontic considerations are excluded from the analysis by interviewing the patient or reading their dental history. In an adult population, it becomes more difficult to determine if missing teeth are due to the results of caries or periodontal disease. The DMF Index is used for permanent teeth and not primary teeth because missing primary teeth may be a result of natural exfoliation or extraction.

The "F" component of the index is indicative of the amount of treatment that has been received as opposed to the "D" component which is indicative of the amount of unmet need. In some situations the "F" component may overrepresent the amount of caries activity that preceded it. For example, a tooth which has been covered by a full crown is counted as five filled surfaces even though fewer surfaces may have been actually carious prior to crown preparation.

The DMF Index is most useful if reported by stratum specific characteristics such as age instead of overall rates for a population. The 1979-80 National Dental Caries Prevalence Survey obtained the following DMFT and DMFS values of children aged 5 to 17. Note that in some cases the standard deviation is larger than the mean. This indicates an asymmetric distribution with a long tail. Preferable descriptors to the mean and standard deviation in this case would be median and range.

TABLE A-1

MEAN DMFT AND DMFS AND STANDARD DEVIATIONS FOR CHILDREN 5-17 YEARS, BOTH SEXES U.S. 1979-1980, ALL REGIONS

Age	Mean DMFT	St. Dev.	Mean DMFS	St. Dev.
5	0.07	0.427	0.11	0.793
6	0.16	0.535	0.20	0.727
7	0.44	0.935	0.58	1.437
8	0.90	1.306	1.25	2.068
9	1.26	1.538	1.90	2.775
10	1.69	1.750	2.60	3.210
11	1.96	1.928	3.00	3.513
12	2.64	2.522	4.18	4.705
13	3.38	2.887	5.41	5.546
14	4.04	3.477	6.53	6.608
15	4.94	3.989	8.07	7.889
16	5.54	4.072	9.58	9.192
17	6.35	4.524	11.04	10.200

References:

Klein, H., Palmer, C.E., Knutson, J.W. "Studies on Dental Caries." I. Dental Status and Dental Needs of Elementary School Children, Public Health Reports, Vol. 53, pp. 751-765, 1938.

Caries Measurement Task Group. Conference on Clinical Testing of Cariostatic Agents, American Dental Association, Chicago, October 14-16, 1968.

Data Processing Manual, Biometry Section, National Caries Program, NIDR, 1975.

National Caries Program, NIDR, The prevalence of dental caries in United States children, 1979-1980. U.S. Dept. H.H.S. NIH Pub. No. 32-2245, pp. 11-12, December, 1981.

THE def AND df INDICES

Because of the difficulty encountered in applying the DMF Index to primary teeth, Gruebbel devised the **def** system to measure the "observable dental caries prevalence" in primary teeth. The "d" represents the number of **decayed primary teeth indicated for filling;** the "e" represents the number of **decayed primary teeth indicated for extraction;** and the "f" represents the number of **filled primary teeth** for each child examined. In this index, the "d" and the "e" both represent teeth that are carious, although with different levels of severity, and teeth that have been extracted due to caries are not represented. Thus, the total caries experience is underestimated. Many investigators combine the "d" and the "e" categories and refer to the **df** index. The df index is less subjective and decreases examiner variability. The denominator of these indices, as in the DMF indices, is the number of children examined.

Reference:

Gruebbel, A.O. A measurement of dental caries prevalence and treatment service for deciduous teeth. J. of Dental Research, Vol. 23, No. 3, pp. 163-168, 1944.

ORAL HYGIENE INDEX

The **Oral Hygiene Index (OHI)** developed by Green and Vermillion is composed of two parts: a **Debris Index (DI)** and a **Calculus Index (CI).** For each of these two components, 12 measurements are recorded, one for the buccal and one for the lingual surface of each of the three segments, one anterior and two posterior, in each arch.

The posterior segments include the teeth distal to the cuspids and the anterior segments include the incisors and cuspids. The score is based on the surface in a particular segment that has the greatest amount of debris, as determined by running an explorer along the sides of the teeth to see how much debris is removed, or the surface that has the greatest amount of calculus, as determined by visual inspection or by probing with the explorer.

The scores and criteria for oral debris and for oral calculus are presented in Tables A2 and A3.

TABLE A-2

	SCORES AND CRITERIA FOR DEBRIS INDEX
Score	Criteria
0	No debris or stain present
1	Soft debris covering not more than one third of the tooth surface being examined or the presence of extrinsic stains without debris regardless of surface area.
2	Soft debris covering more than one third but not more than two thirds of the exposed tooth surface.
3	Soft debris covering more than two thirds of the exposed tooth surface.

TABLE A-3

	SCORES AND CRITERIA FOR CALCULUS INDEX
Score	Criteria
0	No calculus present.
1	Supragingival calculus covering not more than one third of the exposed tooth surface being examined.
2	Supragingival calculus covering more than one third but not more than two thirds of the exposed tooth surface, or the presence of individual flecks of subgingival calculus around cervical portion of the tooth.
3	Supragingival calculus covering more than 2/3 of the exposed tooth surface or a continous heavy band of subgingival calculus around the cervical portion of the tooth.

Thus, in determining the debris or calculus index, each score ranges from 0-3. The sum of the 12 scores ranges from 0-36. The sum of the 12 scores is divided by 6 if 6 segments are being evaluated. If fewer segments are being evaluated, divide by the number of segments included. The maximum score for all six segments is 36/6 = 6.

The Oral Hygiene Index is determined by the summation of the Debris Index and the Calculus Index.

TABLE A-4

SAMPLE RECORDING FORM

DEBRIS						CALCULUS				
	Right	Ant.	Left	Totals			Right	Ant.	Left	Totals
Upper (B) (L)						Upper (B) (L)				
Lower						Lower				
Totals						Totals				

Debris Index = $\dfrac{\text{Total debris score (0-36)}}{\text{\# of Segments scored (0-6)}}$ Calculus Index = $\dfrac{\text{Total calculus score (0-36)}}{\text{\# of segments scored (0-6)}}$

Oral Hygiene Index = Debris Index + Calculus Index

SOURCE: Greene, J.C., Vermillion, J.R. "The oral hygiene index: A method for classifying oral hygine status." J.A.D.A., Vol. 61, August 1960, p. 172-179.

THE SIMPLIFIED ORAL HYGIENE INDEX

The **Simplified Oral Hygiene Index (OHI-S),** has the same criteria for determining tooth surface debris and calculus status as the Oral Hygiene Index. The methodology differs primarily with respect to the number and type of surfaces evaluated. In this simplified version, only six instead of twelve teeth receive scores, one tooth from each of the six segments, and only one surface of each tooth is evaluated. In each of the four posterior segments, the first fully erupted tooth distal to the second bicuspid, usually but not always the first molar, is examined. The buccal surfaces of the maxillary molars and the lingual surfaces of the mandibular molars are scored. In the anterior segments, the buccal surfaces of the upper right and lower left central incisors are scored. The central incisor on the opposite side of the midline can be substituted if the desired anterior tooth is missing.

Since the **Debris Index-Simplified (DI-S)** and **Calculus Index-Simplified (CI-S)** are now based on the sum of 6 scores, each ranging from 0-3, instead of 12 scores, and are still divided by the number of segments, the maximum score for all six segments is 18/6 = 3. The OHI-S score is the sum of DI-S and CI-S and has a range of 0 to 6.

TABLE A-5

Type of Teeth Evaluated	Surface
1 maxillary right molar	buccal
1 maxillary left molar	buccal
1 mandibular right molar	lingual
1 mandibular left molar	lingual
1 maxillary right central incisor	buccal
1 mandibular left central incisor	buccal

Group Index = $\dfrac{\text{sum of individual indexs}}{\text{\# of persons scored}}$

SOURCE: Greene, J.C., Vermillion, J.R. "The simplified oral hygiene index." J.A.D.A., Vol. 68, January, 1964, p.25-31.

THE GINGIVAL INDEX (GI)

The **Gingival Index system (GI)** was developed by Loe and Silness to measure different levels of gingival inflammation. Thus, this index is used to evaluate the gingival tissue for gingivitis and reversible stages of periodontal disease, but does not assess bone loss or irreversible stages of periodontitis. The gingiva around the teeth are examined using a mouth mirror and a periodontal probe to determine changes in color, texture, tendency to hemorrhage and presence or absence of ulceration. The gingiva around all the teeth present may be included in the index, or the index may be limited to the gingiva surrounding the following six teeth:

1) maxillary right first molar
2) maxillary right lateral incisor
3) maxillary left first bicuspid
4) mandibular left first molar
5) mandibular left lateral incisor
6) mandibular right first bicuspid

The gingiva around each tooth is divided into four areas corresponding to the mesial, distal, buccal and lingual surfaces of the tooth. Each of the four areas around each tooth is given a score of 0-3 according to the following criteria.

TABLE A-6

	SCORES AND CRITERIA FOR GINGIVAL INDEX
Score	**Criteria**
0	Absence of inflammation.
1	Mild inflammation — slight change in color and little change in texture.
2	Moderate inflammation — moderate glazing, redness, oedema, and hypertrophy. Bleeding on pressure.
3	Severe inflammation — marked redness and hypertrophy. Tendency to spontaneous bleeding. Ulceration.

The examiner may choose to evaluate only one interproximal surface. If this is done, the interproximal score obtained can be counted twice for inclusion in the index.

The mean of the four scores obtained around each tooth yields the GI for the tooth. The GI scores for all of the teeth examined are summed and divided by the number of teeth examined to obtain the GI for the individual.

References:

Loe, H. and Silness, J. Periodontal disease in pregnancy. I. Prevalence and severity. Acta Odont. Scand., Vol. 21, No. 6, pp. 533-551, 1963.

Loe, H. The gingival index, the plaque index and the retention index systems. J. of Periodontology, Part III, Vol. 38 (supplement), pp. 610-616, 1967.

SULCUS BLEEDING INDEX

The **Sulcus Bleeding Index (SBI)** developed by Muhlemann and Son is similar to the **Gingival index (GI)** but was designed to be more sensitive in its ability to detect early symptoms of gingivitis. This can be an important factor in a short term clinical trial. Results of a study conducted by Muhlemann and Son indicated that bleeding from the gingival sulcus upon gentle probing precedes gingivitis and may occur in gingival areas that have an externally healthy appearance. Thus, the presence or absence of bleeding upon probing is an important criteria in this index.

Muhlemann and Son used eight anterior teeth in each arch, a total of sixteen teeth, in their index methodology. A score is assigned for each of four gingival areas around each tooth, labial and lingual marginal gingival areas and mesial and distal papillary gingival areas, for a total of 64 gingival areas or units per person examined. Each area is gently probed using a blunt periodontal probe with a diameter of .5mm and observed for 30 seconds after probing to detect bleeding. It is necessary to calibrate and standardize examiners so that their functional definition and operation of "gentle probing" is consistent. Generally examiner agreement on the outcome of the probing, presence or absence of bleeding, is easier to obtain than agreement among examiners on other symptoms of periodontal diseases such as presence or absence of color change or edema.

The scoring criteria for the SBI are presented in Table A7 and range from 0 to 5. Results are reported by frequency of each score, mean and standard deviation.

TABLE A-7

SCORES AND CRITERIA FOR SULCUS BLEEDING INDEX

Scores	Criteria
0	Healthy appearance of P and M, not bleeding on sulcus probing
1	Apparently healthy P and M showing no change in color and no swelling, but bleeding from sulcus on probing
2	Bleeding on probing and change of color due to inflammation. No swelling nor macroscopic edema
3	Bleeding on probing and change in color and slight edematous swelling
4	(1) Bleeding on probing and change in color and obvious swelling
5	(2) Bleeding on probing and obvious swelling
	Bleeding on probing and spontaneous bleeding and change in color, marked swelling with or without ulceration.

SOURCE: Muhlemann, H.R., and Son, S. Gingival sulcus bleeding — a leading symptom in intial gingivitis. Helvetia Odent. Acta. 15:107-13, Oct. 1971

Variations of this index include examination of the gingival area surrounding other selected teeth, and reporting only the presence or absence of bleeding on probing.

Reference:

Muhlemann, H.R., and Son, S. Gingival sulcus bleeding - a leading symptom in initial gingivitis. Helvetia Odent. Acta. 15:107-13, October, 1971.

THE PLAQUE INDEX

The **Plaque Index (PlI)** developed by Silness and Loe evaluates the amount of plaque and soft debris located at the gingival margins of the teeth. The absence or presence and quantity of debris is determined both visually and by running a pointed probe across the tooth at the entrance of the gingival crevice. All of the teeth may be included in the evaluation, or the same six teeth that can be selected for the companion gingival index. As in the gingival index, the four gingival areas of each tooth corresponding to the buccal, lingual, mesial and distal surfaces are each given a score ranging from 0 to 3 according to the following criteria.

TABLE A-8

SCORES AND CRITERIA FOR PLAQUE INDEX	
Scores	Criteria
0	No plaque.
1	A film of plaque adhering to the free gingival margin and adjacent area of the tooth. The plaque may be seen *in situ* only after application of disclosing solution or by using the probe on the tooth surface.
2	Moderate accumulation of soft deposits within the gingival pocket, or on the tooth and gingival margin which can be seen with the naked eye.
3	Abundance of soft matter within the gingival pocket and/or on the tooth and gingival margin.

A mean value is obtained based on the four scores for each tooth to obtain the PlI for the tooth. The indices for all of the teeth examined are summed, and divided by the number of teeth examined to obtain the PlI for the individual.

The same recording format presented for the GI can be used for the PlI.

References:

Silness, J. and Loe, H. Periodontal disease in pregnancy, II. Correlation between oral hygiene and periodontal condition. Acta Odont. Scand., Vol. 22, No. 1, pp. 112-135, 1964.

Loe, H. The gingival index, the plaque index and the retention index systems. J. of Periodontology, Part II. Vol. 38 (supplement), pp. 610-616, 1967.

PERIODONTAL DISEASE INDEX

The **Periodontal Disease Index (PDI)** developed by Ramfjord is a combination of a gingivitis score based on the color, form, density and bleeding tendency of gingival tissues and the measurement of pocket depths in relation to the cementum enamel junction (CEJ). The index is based on the following six teeth:

1) maxillary right first molar
2) maxillary left central incisor
3) maxillary left first bicuspid
4) mandibular left first molar
5) mandibular right central incisor
6) mandibular right first bicuspid

The area around each of these teeth should be dried and the gingival health around each tooth scored from 0 to 3 according to the following criteria:

TABLE A-9

SCORES AND CRITERIA FOR GINGIVAL HEALTH STATUS IN PERIODONTAL DISEASE INDEX

Scores	Criteria
0	Absence of inflammation.
1	Mild to moderate inflammatory gingival changes not extending all around the tooth.
2	Mild to moderately severe gingivitis extending all around the tooth.
3	Severe gingivitis characterized by marked redness, tendency to bleed, and ulceration.

Next, pocket depths from the CEJ are determined for the mesial, buccal, distal and lingual aspects of each of the six teeth under evaluation. If the gingival margin is on the enamel, then 1) the distance from the free gingival margin to the cementum enamel junction along each surface is recorded as well as 2) the distance from the free gingival margin to the bottom of the pocket are recorded. Measurement 1 subtracted from measurement 2 yields the desired measurement of the distance from the CEJ to the bottom of the pocket. If the gingival margin is on the cementum, the value from the CEJ to the bottom of the pocket is measured directly.

To determine the periodontal disease score for each tooth, the following system is used:

1) If the gingival sulcus does not extend apically beyond the

CEJ, then the score of 0-3 recorded for the gingival health status is considered the PDI score for the tooth.

2) If the pocket depth extends apically beyond the CEJ, but not by more than 3 mm. along any of the four aspects of the tooth, then a score of 4 is assigned for that tooth.

3) If the gingival crevice extends from more than 3mm. to 6mm. apically from the CEJ, then the tooth receives a score of 5. Finally, if the distance between the CEJ and the bottom of the gingival crevice is more than 6mm. along the root, the tooth receives a score of 6. This system is summarized in the following table:

TABLE A-10

PERIODONTAL DISEASE INDEX SCORES

Location of Gingival Sulcus	Score	Comment
On enamel or at CEJ	0-3	Use gingival health status score
≤ 3mm Apical to CEJ	4	Disregard gingival status score
> 3mm to ≤ 6mm Apical to CEJ	5	Disregard gingival status score
> 6mm Apical to CEJ	6	Disregard gingival status score

SOURCE: Ramfjord, S. Indices for prevalence and incidence of periodontal disease. J of Periodontology, Vol. 30, No. 1, p. 51-59, 1959.

The PDI score for the individual is the mean score for all the teeth examined; the sum of the scores for each tooth examined divided by the number of teeth examined.

This index is more useful when used on an individual basis or for clinical trials than for large-scale population surveys.

Reference:

Ramfjord, S. Indices for prevalence and incidence of periodontal disease. J. of Periodontology, Vol. 30, No. 1, pp. 51-59, 1959.

THE PERIODONTAL INDEX

The **Periodontal Index (PI)** was developed by Russell to be used as an epidemiologic tool to compare the relative prevalence of periodontal disease in different populations. Because it is based on detecting more overt signs of disease, it is not very sensitive and may underestimate early stages of disease. However, because the criteria used are easier to detect, there is less examiner variability and results have good reproducibility. The scoring system is weighted to place more emphasis on more advanced stages of disease.

A mouth mirror and an explorer are used and a good light source is important. Each tooth is assigned a score based on the following criteria used to quantify the health or extent of disease present in the periodontium.

TABLE A-11

SCORES AND CRITERIA FOR PERIODONTAL INDEX

Scores	Criteria
0	Negative. There is neither overt inflammation in the investing tissues nor loss of function due to destruction of supporting tissue.
1	Mild gingivitis. There is an overt area of inflammation in the free gingivitis which does not circumscribe the tooth.
2	Gingivitis. Inflammation completely circumscribes the tooth, but there is no apparent break in the epithelial attachment.
6	Gingivitis with pocket formation. The epithelial attachment has been broken and there is a pocket (nor merely a deepened gingival crevice due to swelling in the free gingivae). There is no interference with normal masticatory function, the tooth is firm in its socket, and has not drifted.
8	Advanced destruction with loss of masticatory function. The tooth may be loose; may have drifted; may sound dull on percussion with a metallic instrument; may be depressible in its socket.

Inflammation, pocket formation, and tooth mobility are all taken into consideration in this index.

The PI score for an individual is the mean score for all the teeth examined. A population score can be computed by obtaining a mean of all the individual scores.

Russell described the relationships that he found between the diagnoses and PI scores that were obtained for a group of 601 Colorado patients in a field setting. These relationships are presented in Table A12. There is considerable overlap of PI scores between clinical diagnoses, especially for less severe disease categories.

TABLE A-12

RELATIONSHIP BETWEEN CLINICAL DIAGNOSES AND PERIODONTAL INDEX SCORES

Diagnosis	68.8% Conf. Interval $\bar{x} \pm 1$ S.D.
Clinically normal supportive tissues	0 - .2
Simple gingivitis	.3 - .9
Beginning destructive periodontal disease	.7 - 1.9
Established destructive periodontal disease	1.6 - 5.0
Terminal disease	3.8 - 8.0

The PI has been used successfully throughout the world under a variety of field conditions.

References:

Russell, A.L. A system of classification and scoring for prevalence surveys of periodontal disease. J. of Dental Research, Vol. 35, No. 3, pp. 350-359, 1956.

Russell, A.L. The periodontal index. J. of Periodontology, Part II. Vol. 38 (supplement), pp. 585-591, 1967.

ORAL HEALTH STATUS INDICES

Nikias, M.K., Sollecito, W.A. and Fink, R. An oral health status index based on ranking of oral status profiles by panels of dental professionals.J. of Public Health Dentistry, Vol. 39, No. 1, pp. 16-26, 1979.

Marcus, M., Koch, A.L. and Gershen, J.A. A proposed index of oral health status: a practical application. J.A.D.A., Vol. 107 pp.729-733, 1983.

INDEX